7.95

D1384333

COMMUNITY DYNAMICS
AND MENTAL HEALTH

Community Dynamics and Mental Health

DONALD C. KLEIN

*Center for Community Affairs,
NTL Institute for Applied Behavioral Science
Washington, D.C.*

JOHN WILEY & SONS, INC.
New York · London · Sydney · Toronto

Library of Congress Catalog Card Number: 68-8105
SBN 471 49050 4
Printed in the United States of America

Foreword

Revolutionary advances in the concepts of mental illness and mental health have brought about the development of new professional roles. Psychiatric concerns of two decades ago centered in mental hospitals. When psychodynamic understanding of medical illness became possible, psychiatrists began to feel at home in general hospitals. Still later, as the social sciences began to offer new understanding of the social order and the human environment of actual and prospective patients, the opportunities for prevention and for effective rehabilitation beckoned psychiatrists into the center of community life.

They soon found that work in the community was full of pitfalls and would lead to rapid discouragement unless psychiatric insights and efforts were blended with the resources being developed in the fields of social psychology, anthropology, sociology, and organization theory. It was necessary to form teams of workers in mental health and social psychiatry in which the skills and the knowledge of these different disciplines were aligned for mutual understanding and for harmonious team play in trying to master some of the most challenging community problems. The center of concern was not the patient but the population of the community, its well-being, its provision for the sick, the disordered, and the disabled, and its own helping resources for safeguarding its members at times of crisis and under the impact of social change.

Much intensive work has taken place during the last two decades to make this kind of collaboration possible. Donald Klein is one of the pioneers who at the beginning of this period stepped into a still novel, uncharted territory. He engaged in the creation of an agency dedicated to and embedded in an expanding suburb at the edge of a metropolis. Much community engineering was required to develop opportunities for research in preventive psychiatry. Patterns of participation with the caretaking professions had to be forged, and the complex interplay of forces contending for goals other than mental health had to be understood. It was necessary to learn by trial and error how the new agency could participate in the solution of problems meaningful to the citizens.

The author's rich experience as executive director of the Wellesley Human Relations Service, compounded with the insight and detailed knowledge of human interaction he acquired from the study of group processes and tested by further experience in consulting on community problems, provides a basis for the formulations presented in this book. He introduces dynamic concepts that allow the reader to discern orderly sequences in community events and to relate them to fruitful methods of intervention.

There is much in this book to stimulate the discussion of theoretical issues. The author has drawn on a wide spectrum of formulations from the behavioral sciences to arrive at a usable conceptual framework. Community problem solving is seen as taking place in the context of integrative forces that may be more easily overlooked than those having to do with conflict and disintegration. The description of the challenge presented to local communities by their embeddedness in and dependence on regional and national bodies is particularly timely.

Dr. Klein never loses sight of the central theme of mental health. He clearly expands its field of endeavor to include not only the well-being of individual members of the community but also the patterns of organization devised to cope with the inevitable crises in community life.

To my knowledge there has not been available until now a clear and concise statement of typical community problems, a useful roster of concepts, and a description of obstacles as well as problem-solving methods. Such a resource is badly needed by the staffs of the emerging community mental health centers. This book will do much to prevent mental health workers from retreating to the safe haven of the traditional clinic by giving them an orderly appraisal, encouraging them to tackle what can be done, and pointing out those problems that may best be left alone until more understanding is achieved.

Most important, however, in my opinion, is the fact that this book circumscribes in a convincing way the emerging field of professional community psychology. It is in this area that the psychologist as participant observer can make indirectly a major contribution to the understanding and mastery of mental illness while he is focusing on being a significant resource in the resolution of community problems and conflicts.

ERICH LINDEMANN

Stanford, California
Spring, 1968

Preface

In this book I have sought to avoid reducing community dynamics to the level of individual and group phenomena. Those trained in mental health are likely to explain community-based behavior as "nothing but" the manifestations of individual needs, conflicts, and defense mechanisms or of group problems having to do with such phenomena as authority, communication, and cohesiveness. To do so, however, is to run the risk of violating the uniqueness of community. It is the kind of interpretation that misses the more fundamental *gestalts* and patterned interactions of community life, which in my opinion transcend the motivations of individuals and the dynamics of face-to-face groups, though by no means excluding them.

There are unique processes of community life—most of which are still poorly defined—that cannot adequately be described in individual, group, or, for that matter, organizational terms. Therefore I have sought to approach the community at a level of magnification appropriate to it. The object has been to keep the power of magnification reduced sufficiently to permit attention to the larger, grosser patterns of community interaction that would not become apparent if more refined analysis were attempted.

The dynamics of conflict, for example, have been treated solely by large-system analysis rather than in intrapsychic or even interpersonal terms. Community action has been viewed somewhat macroscopically as a sequence of steps by which goals become established, responsibilities determined, and action steps located in the larger matrix of the community rather than in terms of the motivational or need systems of the individuals involved.

This book was written to help mental health teams and their many allies to be more effective in their efforts to create community-based mental health programs. You will discover, however, that it has the further objective of fostering creative doubts about the ultimate efficacy of much that passes today for community programming in the field. The chief doubt, shared by many colleagues, concerns the notion that the way to mentally healthy communities is to be found primarily in the institutional hallways of comprehensive mental health centers.

We are accustomed to the cause-effect juxtaposition of means and ends. A nation wishes to achieve the ends of mental health for all its citizens; therefore it establishes the means of trained workers to man specially established facilities and programs. It may help you to understand the book's fundamental bias if I acknowledge at the outset that I no longer accept this simple means-end formulation. I believe that the goal of a mentally healthy society—leaving aside whatever this rhetoric may mean to you, me, or any other set of visionaries—is not the kind of final outcome that can be attained by agencies and programs. Rather it is the kind of objective that is achieved or lost by the very nature of the *processes* by which such agencies and programs are developed. It is the quality of those processes with which I hope you are or will become most concerned. For it is *how* the community goes about meeting problems and making decisions that affects its citizen's social and emotional wellbeing at least as much as, if not more than, the nature of the solutions or decisions.

It is a far cry from a sanitary land-fill system or garbage disposal to the operating amphitheatre of a general hospital. Yet the prevention of physical disease and the maintenance of the community's physical health is more dependent on the former than it is on the latter. This is not to say that a comprehensive community health program does not rest on both. It must, of course. I use the analogy only to underscore the unfortunate fact that in mental health to date we have been far more inclined to stress the specialized, medically based treatment and consulting programs than the more earthy operations of fostering the community mental health equivalents of pure water supplies and adequate garbage disposal.

The book reflects my conviction that it is possible—by the use of community development approaches, techniques of education for both adults and children, and strategies of social intervention—for mental health teams to play their part in making the community a more meaningful environment, socially and emotionally. To do so, however, it is necessary to make one simple but highly significant shift in figure-ground relationship. The community cannot remain only the setting in which the mental health agency operates; instead, it must become the essential source of mental health itself. With this shift in emphasis, the arrangements within the mental health facility itself (assuming there must always be one, which may not necessarily be the case) become secondary to a consideration of the more comprehensive arrangements within the total community by which the safety of the people is assured, their self-development, fostered, and assistance provided when they are in need.

You will find that the book is not a Baedeker of community landmarks and institutions. Rather it offers several different conceptual vantage points from which any community can be viewed, hopefully both with clarity and some purpose. The emphasis is on processes and the interplay of forces. Decision making, communication, linkage, and interdependence within and between communities, change and conflict, action, and, above all, development are the defining attributes of the community's terrain as viewed from the perspectives offered.

Nonetheless, I suppose the book will have an occasional "how to" flavor for some. If so, put it down to the understandable, though perhaps misguided zeal of a consultant who, caught up in his client's goals, could not avoid an occasional, "If I were you, what I would do is. . . ." You may even find such "practical," "down to earth" suggestions the most useful part of the book. If so, fine; for it is probably true that my own experiences are not totally irrelevant as a guide to others. I hope, however, that you will also be challenged and stimulated to acquire increased sensitivity toward and awareness of community phenomena. I hope you will end up by being able to observe the community in new ways and with a richer and more complete cognitive map; that you will think about the community in new ways, and that your appraisals of community situations and events in which you are involved will be better informed than they would have been if neither of us had invested time and effort in these pages. Out of all this I hope will come the insightful advice to yourselves that is usually far more relevant as the basis for effective action or community intervention than is the "how to" advice of others.

This volume is addressed explicitly to mental health workers and students preparing themselves for the field. It talks about mental health issues and draws most of its examples from that field. I confess, however, that I wrote it with the hope that it might also serve a wider audience. In fact, at the suggestion of adult educator Malcolm Knowles I used the device of addressing myself to six good friends deliberately chosen from differing backgrounds. I tried to write in a manner that would do justice to their varied disciplines and experiences, with the hope that they might profit from having read it.

I started with Malcolm himself. The other five were one of the graduate fellows in the community psychology program at Boston University, a psychoanalyst director of a community psychiatry training center, a sociologist who specializes in the American community, the president of a state chapter of the League of Women Voters, and an expert consultant in the field of community development.

To the extent that I succeeded in my purpose the book will serve a wider group that numbers all those whose efforts are helping to shape tomorrow's communities. Among them are the many civic leaders involved in voluntary associations for mental health and other areas of community betterment; elected and appointed government officials, including those working in such critical areas as housing and urban renewal, law enforcement and civil rights, and the war on poverty, as well as education, health, and welfare; community development specialists; social workers in community organization, group work, and agency administration; physical and social planners; educators of adults as well as children; and the growing body of applied behavioral scientists (from sociology, anthropology, psychology, and other disciplines) for whom the application of the knowledge of human behavior is an intrinsic part of the process by which such knowledge becomes fully developed.

Because the book draws from many fields, it very likely does justice to none. It may be open to criticism of partial coverage from specialists in all the areas from which it borrows. I have no defense against such criticism except to point out that the book is an attempt to form an *amalgam* of several elements rather than to set forth the essential nature of any one. The main concern must come, I believe, at those points at which the result has been more a juxtaposition than a blending. If you find that the attempted amalgam does not succeed for you, it is either because the elements are inherently recalcitrant and resist unification or because as an intellectual centrifuge I leave something to be desired.

DONALD C. KLEIN

Washington, D.C.
June 1968

Acknowledgments

This volume's approach to community dynamics has developed from an assortment of significant encounters with individuals and their ideas, with institutions, and with communities. The chief contributors during ten years with the mental health program in Wellesley were Dr. Erich Lindemann and his wife Elizabeth, the latter one of the most competent community consultants I have known. Dr. Gerald Caplan provided new insights into the dynamics of the consulting process. Others on the Wellesley staff for whose influence I am grateful are sociologist Dr. A. Paul Hare, social psychologist Dr. Clara Mayo, social workers Lois Paul, Marie McNabola, and Dr. William Freeman, and psychologists Dr. Pearl Rosenberg and Dr. John von Felsinger. Citizens, too, added much to my understanding of community. Among them I think of the Reverend Dr. William Rice, Reverend John Wallace, Curtis Hilliard, Marion Niles, Katharine Bronson, John Chaffee, Richard Viguers, Albert and Jessie Danielsen, Violet Goodrich, and Betty Farley. The list is far too long to complete and I am certain to have slighted many who contributed to my education.

A program grant from the National Institute of Mental Health to the Department of Psychiatry, Massachusetts General Hospital, made it possible to convene in 1960 a continuing workshop on community processes during which many of the ideas presented in this book were developed or sharpened. Many colleagues contributed. I recall especially Dr. von Felsinger, Dr. Wesley Allinsmith, Doris Fraser, Dr. Louisa Howe, Dr. James Kelly, Dr. Robert Newbrough, Virginia Sachs, and Dr. Alvin Simmons.

As a byproduct of the workshop there began a three-year collaboration with Laura Morris, social worker, and Dr. Fred Duhl, psychiatrist, during which time we developed an outline for a book and I wrote drafts of several chapters. Though I cannot ask either Laura or Fred to assume responsibility for this volume's limitations, it would not have been written without them and I hope they will see some of their influence reflected in its pages.

Epidemiologists Dr. Frank Babbott and Dr. Brian McMahon at the Harvard School of Public Health contributed to my knowledge of their field. Colleagues within the National Training Laboratories in several ways have extended my understanding of community dynamics beyond the confines of mental health. Probably the most influential conceptual impacts have been made in community sociology by Dr. Edward Moe and Dr. Roland Warren and in community development by Dr. Richard Franklin and H. Curtis Mial.

At Boston University the Human Relations Center provided a unique and exciting setting within which to absorb and practice theories and approaches to community change as stated and applied with the greatest impact for me by Drs. Kenneth Benne and Robert Chin.

The list of experiences, settings, and individuals who have helped fashion the material of this volume also includes my mother and father who modeled in their lives a sense of civic responsibility and participation. For them the question was never *whether* to be involved, only *how*. Rabbi Levi Olan and religious youth director William Fury of Temple Emanuel in Worcester, Massachusetts, contributed a yeasty concern for social issues. Finally, I am grateful to my wife Lola who, on the basis of her unique childhood experiences in a progressive community and school atmosphere, has helped me to re-examine many of my assumptions about community institutions and processes.

The book was completed because of the generous editorial assistance and typing efforts of others. Ilene Herson and Harry Hollander worked diligently on the initial bibliography; sections of the first draft were prepared by Ilene, Susan Salsburg and Nora Ginman; Miriam Freedman worked long and conscientiously on the typing of the final manuscript assisted by Diann Birdsong, Joan Kieff, Dawn Patten, and Virginia Stacy. Additional bibliographic references were provided by Robert Luke, Jr., and his wife Barbara. The initial index was prepared by Elizabeth Uprichard. Robert Luke, Curtis and Dorothy Mial, Drs. Eugene Long, Hans Spiegel, and Leonard Hassol, and my wife Lola offered frank and searching editorial criticisms and suggestions. Mimeographing and final assembly of the manuscript were carried out by Donald Rankin, who put in many overtime hours to see the job through in time. Typing of final revisions was done by Carlotta Dabney.

D. C. K.

Contents

of Responsibilities by Big Government, Membership in Vertical Associations, Social Planning

COMMUNITY DYNAMICS
AND MENTAL HEALTH

1

The Community as a Setting for Mental Health Work

"A community is basically an educational medium, whatever other purpose its parts may serve. What kinds of people does it produce? In the answer to this question lies the moral, the human criterion of its maturity or immaturity, its excellence or its disgrace."

KENNETH BENNE, *Criteria of a Mature Community.*

CHAPTER ONE

A Mental Health Definition of Community

For years people entering mental hospitals and clinics checked their communities at the door. Fortunately, in most places this state of affairs is rapidly changing and we are, as one of the leaders in the field has put it, beyond "the point of no return in our long journey from a helter-skelter system . . . either divorced from community life or at least not geared to it" (Felix, 1964, p. 1809). As of June 30, 1967, after two years under the federal grants program, 256 community mental health centers had been funded. One hundred thirty million dollars had been allocated for construction, staffing, or both. The centers are located in forty-eight states, the District of Columbia, and Puerto Rico, and will serve forty-one million people in rural areas, suburbia, and the core city (Yolles, 1967). If present plans are implemented, all the afore-mentioned is merely a beginning; moreover, these figures do not take into account existing clinics and other mental health activities funded by mental health associations and other means.

Now that the quest is on for effective means of preventing psycholog-ical problems and promoting psychological soundness, there is growing recognition of a need to understand and use community forces in the pursuit of mental health. We are in the midst of a virtual about face in the orientation of an entire field. As a result, mental health programs all over the country are confronting communities in new ways. This, in turn, requires more attention to the nature and meaning of community life and new attempts to understand the basic dynamics of the com-munity.

It also requires a new look at what is meant by mental health and how, if at all, mental health and the community are interrelated. An an-swer to this question requires some attention first to what is meant by

3

health. We know that health is usually viewed as an attribute of the individual. Moreover, most experts conclude that health fundamentally represents a conclusion about the physical or psychological status of the individual, heavily loaded with the values and biases of the culture (Jahoda, 1958; J. Clausen, 1963). Especially insofar as medicine has turned its attention to public health, preventive medicine, and, more recently, psychiatry, it has accepted a holistic frame of reference in which psychological, social, and cultural aspects are related to both man's biology and his environment (Straus and Clausen, 1963). Probably all that can be agreed on is that health is an absence of disease. Beyond this it is basically the culture's decision whether to place a high value on such characteristics as flexibility or rigidity, introversion or extroversion, emotional lability or emotional control, passivity or aggressivity. To be sure, the criteria of reality testing and, more recently, social competence (L. Phillips, 1967) are sometimes offered as ways out of the value dilemma. However, the realities with which any individual copes are complex and shifting and the realities for different individuals are often not alike, especially when the individuals come from vastly different cultural or socioeconomic backgrounds. We can agree that adequate reality testing is important, but who is to determine which of the several available levels of reality should have priority? Social competence is by definition culture-bound and has the merit of putting mental health in a psychosocial context. It is, in part, the degree to which a person, according to his age and sex, learns to cope effectively with societal expectations (L. Phillips, 1967). Perhaps there is a kind of general social competence factor that underlies man's effectiveness in dealing with the widely varying expectations of different cultures. If so, it is yet to be proved. If such a factor exists, we may be able to concentrate on the social competence of the individual as in the past we have thought of mental health in individual terms. I doubt the wisdom of such an approach, however, for there are some cultures having elements of totalitarianism, war, and poverty, in which it may not be "well" to be socially competent.

THE IMPORTANCE OF COMMUNITY
TO MENTAL HEALTH

In thinking my own way through the problem, I have found that it was diminished, though hardly eliminated, when mental health was defined in terms of social aggregates rather than individuals. I have come to believe that the community represents the single most important social matrix which man has invented and that it is upon this matrix that the concept of mental health can be developed most fruitfully. *In the community one finds all the manifold challenges that confront each one of us as he lives out his life in the company of others who are important to him. The community is the means whereby society imposes its expectations on the person.*

The emotional hazards of life found in the community challenge our adaptive resources and those of the groups in which we live. By definition, an emotional hazard is a circumstance faced by many people in the ordinary course of living which makes demands that are not readily coped with by the mechanisms the individual is accustomed to using. Whatever their nature (e.g., the loss or formation of relationships, adjustment to new settings, or the assumption of new roles or status within the same setting), they represent marked shifts in the equilibrium between an individual and his immediate and most relevant social environment. This environment may consist of a small face-to-face group, a neighborhood, organization, or other social aggregate; but whatever its size and complexity, *that environment which impinges directly on the individual is part of, is maintained by, contributes to, and takes its essential characteristics from, the community.*

Emotional hazards confront large numbers of individuals, but only a few show marked crisis and prolonged disequilibrium. It is apparent that individuals vary in their generalized capacity to deal with emotionally hazardous situations as well as in their competence to deal with specific types of hazards. The immediate emotional well-being of any individual is a function of the nature of the demands made on him and his ability to deal with them. It is also influenced by the environmental supports available to him at times of stress. Once again the community becomes important, for *it is only through the associations and institutions of the community that essential interpersonal and institutional supports become accessible.*

As we direct our thinking away from the more limited concept of mental health as a strictly intra-individual state of affairs, we inevitably become caught up in the quest for understanding of the community as the entity that gives rise both to the hazards of living and to the potentials for coping successfully with them. This conceptualization of mental health and community is neither new nor original. Lindemann (1944), for one, articulated it as the result of his experiences with the delayed recovery from burns and injuries of survivors who had lost loved ones in the Coconut Grove nightclub fire in Boston. Programmatically, the concept is finding its expression in experimentation with comprehensive programs of community mental health, encompassing preventive efforts and promotion of psychological soundness, early intervention at times of crisis to forestall more serious difficulties, and rehabilitation programs for those in need of long-term or continuing care with crippling disorders (Caplan, 1964). It is clear that none of these programs can proceed successfully without attention to the dynamics of community interaction. In each instance the strategy of intervention involves efforts to influence the community, although it does not appear that those manning the programs are always fully aware of the far-reaching community implications of their efforts.

Rehabilitation of former mental patients, for instance, is not achieved by developing posthospitalization clinics and other follow-up services. It will be successful in the final analysis when there is a community that accepts the person as a valued, if not fully functioning, member or citizen. Early interventions and walk-in clinics can be carried out to their ultimate objective of case finding and prompt help only when community resources are mobilized to direct those in need to the available help promptly enough to make it truly effective. Most of all, the community in virtually all its facets becomes implicated when we begin to consider how best to achieve even a semblance of primary prevention and promotion of psychological soundness among large numbers of people. In mental health's current revolution, when it embraced the concepts and approaches of public health, it also, perforce, took on all aspects of the community and its processes (N. Hobbs, 1964).

The fundamental strategy of primary prevention is disarmingly simple. It involves the modification or elimination of the hazard itself or the provision of adequate safeguards so that those exposed to the hazard can cope with it successfully. To set about achieving these objectives, we are confronted with the necessity of understanding and modifying the institutions, orientations, and help giving patterns of the community. Significant programs of prevention and promotion can only be carried out on a community-wide basis. This is obviously true for physical health, which rests as much on the availability of pure drinking water as it does on medical care and treatment of the individual; it is probably equally true for mental health, which, in turn, must be pursued with the impetus of broad social concern and community involvement.

The idea of altering community patterns is staggering when one considers the complexity of what is being altered. By complexity I am not referring primarily to the number of people, heterogeneity of population, intricate network of streets, buildings, and other complex physical and other demographic features. What brings the people together in the first place, keeps them there, and produces the enormous diversity of physical and social features are the varied and essential *functions* performed by the community.

COMMUNITY FUNCTIONS

What are the major functions of the community? There are, of course, some apparent basics, such as:

1. Providing and distributing living space and shelter and determining use of space for other purposes;

2. Making available the means for distribution of necessary goods and services;

3. Maintaining safety and order, and facilitating the resolution of conflicts.

4. Educating and acculturating newcomers (e.g., children and immigrants) ;

5. Transmitting information, ideas, and beliefs;

6. Creating and enforcing rules and standards of belief and behavior;

7. Providing opportunities for interaction between individuals and groups.

The community establishes patterns for such interactions, which rest on differentiation of roles, allocation of social status, and the provision of acceptable means for social mobility.[1]

It seems apparent that the ways in which such functions are handled will have significant implications for psychological well-being. Marginal people, with respect to shelter, social acceptance, or status, will have psychological problems different from those who are not. Those living in situations where conflicts are resolved by violence will differ in perceptions and behavior patterns from those living where no behavioral outlets for hostile feelings are provided. Recent civil rights controversies demonstrate vividly how different are the psychological worlds occupied by the establishment (the opinion shapers and rule makers) and those upon whom rules are enforced and who feel alienated from the sources of power.

[1] A very similar list of community functions has been put forward by Sanders (1958, p. 345), a sociologist: (a) recruitment of new members; (b) communication; (c) differentiation and status allocation; (d) allocation of goods and services; (e) socialization; (f) social control (allocation of power) ; (g) allocation of prestige; (h) social mobility; (i) integration through adjustment (internal accommodation and adjustment to forces outside the system) .

All seven of the above functions are implicated both at the time a mental health facility is established and throughout its existence. How is this so? Let us look briefly at some ways in which the first few functions might become involved just to get a feel for the interplay of community forces in any mental health program:

PROVIDING AND DISTRIBUTING SPACE

The center must be located spatially within the community and decisions made about the kind and amount of space it will occupy. Questions of zoning, land use, property values, and the like are implicitly involved, whether or not they are raised explicitly. Desirable space is not unlimited and there is bound to be open or covert contention about the use of space for mental health as opposed to other purposes.

MAKING AVAILABLE GOODS AND SERVICES

In comparison with other goods and services for which funds and human energies must be spent, how vital is the mental health facility? For the professionals involved and their citizen supporters, it may have a priority well above most other institutions and their needs. Others will not necessarily agree. The establishment of a mental health facility affects all other goods and services to some extent; in addition to the siphoning off of scarce resources, the mental health facility may well materially affect how education, family case work, law enforcement, and a myriad of other functions are handled in the community. The goods and services of the entire community will not be the same as they were before if the mental health center is successful. Thus the decision within the community to create and support the mental health program can be made only when enough people who value other goods and services are convinced that the new facility poses no fundamental threat and, even better, will contribute to the causes in which they are invested.

MAINTAINING SAFETY AND ORDER

Questions of safety and order often arise in connection with mental health projects. Part of the impetus for the mental health program in Wellesley, Massachusetts, for example, came from an apparent rise in juvenile acting-out behavior. Mental health proponents there and elsewhere have had to confront community anxieties over the possibility that their work would unleash aggressivity or sexual aberrations.

Similarly, the potential, if not actual, impact of the mental health field for education, creating and transmitting beliefs, values, and rules is great, though not always so immediately apparent. It brings to the community a definite set of normative assumptions and values about ideal behavior and relations between individuals. When translated into law, as in the Supreme Court school desegregation decision of 1954, these values can have immediate and far-reaching consequences. Consider, for example, the potential effects of the mental health field's orientation toward conflict resolution, an orientation that is grounded in a rich history of work with intrapsychic and interpersonal conflicts and their consequences.

In a project involving several political factions of a city with a mental health team in an attempt to train indigenous nonprofessional community facilitators to work with new neighborhood improvement associations, differences developed between a mental health staff member and an administrator appointed originally by one of the factions. The mental health worker's inclination was to bring together the several individuals involved to bring the problems out into the open in order to diagnose them more adequately and work them through. The administrator and his boss, however, viewed this step as politically naive, at best, and destructive to the integrity and effectiveness of the project, at worst. When the worker pressed his point of view, the rift deepened to the point where it was no longer possible for the administrator and his boss to trust the worker and he was forced to withdraw from the project.

Brought into a community controversy, I and other mental health workers are apt, as a result of our training and experiences, to invite protagonists to consider their motivations or seek ways of reducing interpersonal threat and antagonism. I find I am also disinclined to encourage continued battling about beliefs, principles, or points of view. Initially, at least, I and people like me did not bring much awareness of or comfort with the possibilities for tradeoff, compromise, and political accommodation, which traditionally play a major part in community conflict resolution. I have found also that we are usually concerned that our responsibility to the entire community might be impaired by becoming vigorous fighters for any good cause. It is likely that the inculcation of mental health values and approaches into the community in any large-scale fashion would result in dampening of controversy, reduction of frankly political approaches to the determination of outcomes, and increased recourse to psychological approaches to understanding and managing conflict. I am not suggesting that such an outcome would be unfortunate; I am sure, however, that many people would consider it so. The reader himself can probably go on, if he wishes, to identify other ways in which the mental health center affects community functions, such as the impact on education and socialization it has already had as a result of its humanistic and developmental emphases.

AN INTERACTIONAL DEFINITION
OF COMMUNITY

The identification of the preceding community functions and the analysis of their relevance to community mental health operations go only part of the way toward a statement that would account for the significance of the community to the mental health of its population. For one thing, the functions are stated at different levels of abstraction. Although they serve to call attention to significant areas, they serve mainly as rather large pigeonholes into which a great diversity of community events can be sorted. For another, there is no systematic way in which to account for interrelations between them or to explain why one function becomes operative in certain instances and not others.

Perhaps most important of all, the functions are stated largely from the perspective of the social organizations and their activities (e.g., goods and services equal business and professions; safety and order equal law enforcement; educating newcomers equals public and private schools, etc.) .

Therefore, I have sought a view of community that would simultaneously consist of fewer and less discrete elements, account more adequately for transactions between individuals and social groupings, and have more apparent linkage with what is known about individual and group psychology. I have come up with a tentative statement that continues to be functional in orientation and remains in that tradition of community analysis. It is strongly influenced, however, by interpersonal theories in psychology and the position that mental health practice and research in the community should focus attention on the interactions between individuals and social organizations (Glidewell, 1966) .

Some time ago it occurred to me that virtually all behavior within the community could be boiled down to only a few critical concerns. The first of these has to do with the maintenance of the physical and social environment. The second has to do with finding help and support at times of stress, alluded to earlier in the discussion of emotional hazards. The third has to do with the ways in which individuals gain a sense of self and social worth.

Some time later it became clear that the seven functions listed earlier can be encompassed within a framework provided by the preceding three concerns. Some, like the distribution of goods and services, seem to be concerned primarily with safety and security. Others, such as establishing patterns for interaction between individuals and groups, are concerned with all three. By now, I have reached a point where the very definition of community itself seems to me to rest on a recognition of the importance and prevalence of the three basic concerns.

Any definitional statements about the nature of community face certain dilemmas. One is that, although the most obvious communities are located geographically and represent a concentration of people, other communities (e.g., Jews and Armenians who have lost their homelands) maintain themselves despite the absence of physical locus. Another is that physically based concentrations of population differ radically from one another in the extent to which they are communal (in the sense of sharing any commitment to a common identity or destiny). For example, the "community-ness" of a dispersed metropolitan area, such as Los Angeles, is likely to be far less than that of a more clearly defined, concentrated, and stable area, such as Salt Lake City.[2] Therefore a definition of community, to be most useful, should be applicable to both physically located communities and those that do not depend on physical locus. It should also suggest some ways in which aggregates of people can be differentiated from each other as having more or less of those qualities which make them community.

The community, as I now see it, may be defined as *patterned interactions within a domain of individuals seeking to achieve security and physical safety, to derive support at times of stress, and to gain selfhood and significance throughout the life cycle.* The definition rests on interactions of individuals rather than on the social organizations whose nature and functions are a manifestation of those interactions. The term domain is used to refer both to a physical place that can be geographically located and to a social-psychological place (such as a community of interest) that is *phenomenologically real* to those who inhabit it. The view of community on which this book is based is not that community is man's habitat. Rather, community is man *in* habitat, for the habitat is not meaningful without its inhabitants. Although this distinction is not always made explicit throughout this book, it is present and has affected the selection of material and the emphasis given to it. The remainder of this chapter attempts to clarify the approach, to indicate its relevance to later sections of the book, and to underscore some general implications for the mental health field.

---

2 The manifold problems of developing viable community groupings in urban-metropolitan settings are well delineated in Duhl (1963).

COMMUNITY AND SECURITY

Most communities in this and other industrialized countries are a far cry from the lonely enclaves, tribal gathering places, stockaded towns, and walled feudal domains that are the communities of other times or places. Nonetheless, every community remains physically or psychologically the "huddling place" wherein some semblance of safety and basic security are to be found. Remove community and you have stripped the individual of all the goods and services, common values and beliefs, protective laws, customs, and their enforcers. Leave the individual to exist only within the family or other small primary group, and there is little left but danger and the threat of total destruction.

Most forms of disturbance to the serenity and stability of community produce shock, outrage, and other symptoms of alarm. Outbreaks of crime, major fires, certain strikes, riots, and other civil disturbances are all threats to the sense of security and safety to which man clings precariously through his community. Less obvious but equally threatening for some are violations of codes of belief and behavior, such as unusual dress, hair style, and so-called obscene language. Perhaps because it is the most primary of the three, the aspect of safety or security becomes most apparent only when there is threat to it. At other times it is taken more or less for granted. This is similar to the place accorded physical factors by psychogenic explanations of emotional disorders, which assume that the individual was adequately fed, sheltered, and protected from those noxious physical agents that might have impaired his psychological soundness.

Chapter Four takes up some of the intricacies of such community processes as communication and decision making. They are discussed within the somewhat abstract framework of social system analysis; nonetheless, they can be fully understood only if one accepts the fundamental premise that much of the impetus for both, and therefore much of the alarm which arises when either becomes impaired, comes from the elemental aspect of the community as a huddling place against danger with which the individual alone is unable to deal.

Similar assumptions can be made about community change discussed in Section 4 for it is in connection with change that the pungent fear of danger to community stability, always lurking below the tranquil surface, operates most dramatically. When change agents (from mental health or any other movement) seek to introduce new elements into community life that would alter relationships or modify social custom and law, the elemental fear of threat to safety and security is activated, sometimes intensely and often quite irrationally. The resulting resistance to change serves as a kind of defense, equivalent in many ways to defense mechanisms for the individual. In the former instance, the defense is concerned with the maintenance of the self against the inroads of unacceptable inner impulses and external demands. Resistance at the community level is easily aroused when people are faced with an intrusion of alien and not easily understood forces in the form of ideas, people, or organizations, such as a community mental health agency, a group advocating the religious use of LSD, or newcomers who are different in race, religion, nationality, or some other characteristic.

COMMUNITY AND SUPPORT DURING STRESS

As noted earlier, the community is the setting for a variety of emotional hazards to which all persons are exposed during their lifetimes. Unexpected disruptions, such as those occasioned by accident and illness, loss of loved ones, changes in social role and status, and shifts in relationship occasioned by such events as marriage, change in residence, and birth of a baby, are all times when individuals experience heightened tension, feelings of malaise, and uncertainties, resulting from disruption of familiar patterns and the inadequacy of usual means of coping. Certain hazards, such as the impact on families of birth, bereavement, and marriage, are familiar and repetitive from generation to generation. Because they affect everyone, they have become ritualized within the community through special rites and sacraments. The responsibility to preside over such rituals and to offer support to those involved is given to certain professional groups such as clergymen and physicians. Whether or not rituals are available, the individual facing any hazard is dependent on the resources that a particular community has to offer and is affected by the means of coping that the community either makes available to him or denies him.

The concepts of "crisis theory" and their implications for preventively oriented programming in community mental health have gained great acceptance in recent years (Parad, 1965). The pioneering work of Lindemann (1953, 1956) and Leighton (1959), among others, has developed the perspective presented here, which conceives of the community as the most fundamental matrix within which individuals deal with emotional hazards through a complex pattern of caretaking institutions and individuals.

The earliest, and in many ways the fullest, expression of crisis theory in action was the Human Relations Service of Wellesley, Inc. (Bragg et al., 1958; Naegele, 1955), the pioneer community mental health program initiated by Lindemann in 1948, carried out under the auspices of the Harvard School of Public Health with financing by the W. T. Grant Foundation until 1953, and with local community funding until the present time. Much of the material in this volume is drawn from the Wellesley experience and the rich conceptual framework developed there by Lindemann and his co-workers from public health, behavioral science, and mental health disciplines.

Lindemann viewed the community as the location having the greatest potential for providing supportive resources to individuals. This attitude is reflected both in his writings and in the collaborative way in which he sought to involve local citizens in all aspects of the Wellesley project. Section 3 describes how this view of the community as a primary source of supportive resources shaped the Wellesley experience.

Leighton and his colleagues did comparative studies of small Canadian communities which differed from one another in the extent to which their inhabitants appeared to have cohesiveness, high morale, and mutual regard (Hughes et al., 1960). More highly integrated communities had less delinquency and other social pathology than more poorly integrated ones. This work is reviewed in more detail in the discussion of integrative patterns in Chapter Sixteen.

For now it is enough to note that during times of emotional hazard and individual crisis, disintegrated communities appear to provide fewer and less certain means for problem solving and support than do more integrated ones, either informally via friends and neighbors, or more formally via agencies and professional caretakers.

COMMUNITY AND SELFHOOD

Identification with community affords the individual a sense of having welded the self into an identity that both transcends the person and gives him a worth greater than any he might achieve alone.

The individual's sense of self is shaped both by his communities and his position within them. For mental health purposes, for example, we can draw certain additional inferences from the fact that an individual is not only resident in a certain town but is also employed as a personnel man in a particular company. For we have identified at least two additional communities which may contribute to his sense of self—his company and his profession. If we also learn that he is a newcomer to the town and an officer in the State Society of Training Directors, we now have qualitatively different information bearing on *how he may be viewed in each*. Thus the various roles occupied by an individual reflect both the communities which contribute to his selfhood and the *significance* enjoyed by the person within those communities.

Significance, as it is used here, refers to the value placed on the person by key people in his environment. It is related to, but not synonymous with, self-esteem. The latter refers to the way the individual views himself; the former to the way he is viewed by others. *Sense of significance,* then, becomes the individual's own perception of how he is valued by others. Despite obvious correlation between self-esteem and sense of significance, it is quite possible for one to be high while the other remains low. An example would be an individual with low esteem who loses himself in a cause (e.g., an emotionally unstable soldier who gains a new sense of reflected value among his fellows in a unit with high *esprit de corps*) and finds new significance because of the value placed on him by those with whom he has closed ranks.

Significance may have special value as a concept around which to organize preventively oriented mental health efforts. It is clear that significance in our society is all too frequently interrelated with economic achievement. The poor therefore are rarely permitted significance in the eyes of the wider community (Riessman et al., 1964). Data now available make it clear that such reduced significance can be psychologically disabling over the longrun. Chronically unemployed men studied during the depression of the 1930's showed marked reductions in self-esteem (Hill, 1949); similar problems have been observed among male Negro-Americans (Liebow, 1966) and among immigrant white males from peasant backgrounds whose education and experience made them less able than their wives to adapt to American culture.

Liebow especially has provided a poignant phenomenologic or from the inside-out view of what it is like for rootless men to live a life of insignificance on the streetcorner of a large city. These men, to whom he related for a year, are severely handicapped by lack of money, education, and skills. They move in a traditionless limbo—not quite derelicts or bums; not part either of the stable world of the working man who has a steady job and some faith in what the future may hold for him. They not only are losers; they *know* they are. Their only source of significance is temporary associations with women or fellow losers on the streetcorner—that most inadequate sanctuary which is neither safe, secure, nor satisfying.

Just as psychotherapy for the individual appears to be the method of choice for intervening in emotional disorders marked by impaired self-esteem, intervention in larger social systems would seem to have the greatest promise for enhancing the significance of larger numbers of people and thereby for reducing the incidence of new cases requiring treatment. On a smaller scale, very similar premises have shaped the efforts of those who have sought to transform mental hospitals into self-restorative communities (Jones, 1953). Far more data are needed about the mechanisms whereby individuals are accorded significance, the consequences to both the individual and the community of reliance on each mechanism, and the extent and nature of the ultimate effects on self-esteem of variations of significance level.

MENTAL HEALTH IMPLICATIONS OF AN INTERACTIONAL VIEW

If he views the community as an interactive domain wherein individuals search with greater or lesser success for security, support, and significance, the mental health worker can no longer avoid a deep and abiding interest in the processes of community life. Some of these processes directly affect the welfare of his own mental health facility. That health facility, in turn, becomes a location from which the worker can proceed to discover how his skills can best be used to enhance the community's effectiveness as a source of security, support, and significance for its population.

Having accepted the definition, the worker looks to the community as the social environment in which hazards are experienced and in which supports are provided. He is concerned with how the community determines the kinds of help available at times of stress. He looks into whether such help is sought or offered and, if so, how. He operates on the premise that communities can be influenced to provide more healthy environments and supports that will contribute to the growth and development of their inhabitants. He begins, indeed, with the coordination of efforts within his own domain by providing a continuum of care that embraces in-patient and out-patient care, consultation and other preventive activities, day care and emergency night service, education, and research (Yolles, 1964).

To the extent that the mental health field becomes committed to promoting communities that are suited to the emotional needs of man, its exponents must study the community, immerse themselves in its dynamics, and function ever more effectively as agents of community change. In order to achieve these purposes it is important that mental health workers develop a practical view of community organization—how decisions are made, funds allocated, and new programs initiated and supported. Without the ability to enter into effective partnership with professional and lay leadership, the mental health worker will be stymied at the outset.

With mental health programs being established in communities across the nation, it is important that the professional people involved culti-vate a deep appreciation for the existing patterns of community life and the functions they perform, however inadequately. Succeeding chapters of this book seek to help develop a sense of community based on under-standing of the nature of its complexities and the interdependence of all its aspects. With such understanding we should be able to collaborate with local citizens in bringing about changes that will augment and strengthen community integration and to avoid weakening and disrupt-ing existing resources.

In summary, then, this book is committed to the proposition that people in the mental health field orient themselves to the study of the community for three reasons:

1. To understand the hazards and supports afforded by the social envi-ronment;

2. To learn to work collaboratively with lay and professional citizen groups;

3. To develop approaches which will help create healthier communi-ties that meet human needs more adequately and will avoid inadvertent disruption of community life.

It is hoped that the reader will find this book of some assistance in his quest to understand and work competently and with compassion in community settings.

CHAPTER TWO

The Mental Health Worker's
Sense of Community

When a mental health worker moves into the community, what assumptions does he make and what understandings does he have about the community and his new professional role? What does "community" really mean to him? What *should* it mean?

We have seen that the community, even in today's world of rapid mobility and urban sprawl, is a highly important habitat of man. For it is through the community that man is fed and housed, seeks work, educates his children, and in a myriad of ways maintains his safety and security. It is also through the community that man discovers problems and their solutions, finds spiritual sustenance, exercises his desire for significant participation in life, and occasionally achieves the highest levels of self-actualization and fulfillment.

NEGLECT OF THE COMMUNITY

Yet it is curious that, despite its significance, the community itself as a social matrix has been the subject of relatively little study by the mental health field until the decades following World War II. Unlike the family, which has long featured prominently in our understanding of personality development and character formation, the community until recent years by comparison had been neglected by mental health. Why was this so?

No doubt there are many historic factors, among them the necessary concentration on the nuclear family (a comparatively recent human invention), the growing emphasis on the individual in a technological age, and the erosion of community stability by such factors as the population explosion, geographic mobility, and the like. A related factor is that the mental health worker himself is a creature of the community; it is his habitat, too. He may move through it with no more awareness of its properties than any other person, draw sustenance from it with no more recognition of its importance, and make use of its resources with no greater sense of his dependence on its provision of them.

Indeed, many of us trained in psychiatry, psychiatric social work, and clinical psychology will enter the community mental health field with a less well developed awareness of these matters than the average citizen. We have devoted years of training and practice to intervening with individuals, or at most, family groupings. We have deliberately and for psychotherapeutic reasons dealt with them in settings that have been as removed as possible from their home milieu.

Much of our training has taken place at universities, hospitals, and other settings that in most instances are relatively isolated from other institutions. We may even have lost whatever sense of the local community we once possessed. Most of us no longer are "locals"; our identities are not inextricably interwoven with a single city or town. Instead we are "cosmopolitans"; we identify more closely with those who have the same level of education and the same brand of professional training than we do with the other residents of whatever locality we inhabit. If anything, we tend to avoid involvement in community affairs even when issues affecting us and our families arise.

For some, the prolonged separation or alienation from community affairs may have been sufficient to cause some discomfort during a period of adjustment to the community milieu. Encounters with authority figures—police officers, educators, government officials, social agency workers—from the worker's past may invoke unresolved emotions and conflicts or summon up stereotypes about those groups who are typically known to the small child only as fantasy figures. The child may never have interacted with the school superintendent or police chief in fact; in fantasy, however, either or both may have been potent figures. It can be a startling experience to discover that the bogeyman of the past is in one's present reality simply an individual seeking help or perhaps defending himself against the powerful magic of psychiatry.

There are other problems of transition occasioned by the worker's move into the community (e.g., mental health professionals are typically schooled in a role stance of helper, which requires that someone else present himself in the complementary position of the person seeking help). Many encounters in the community refuse to be shaped according to the rules of the helping game. If the mental health worker is not aware of his predisposition to reinforce tendencies toward establishing helping relationships, he may tend to put on guard and alienate those not willing to fit the pattern.

Mental health workers new to the community often go through a period in which the limits and, in fact, the very nature of their expertise are uncertain and confused. What is their competence if people are not patients? To what extent can the knowledge of human pathology be usefully applied to the management of the range of human problems to be found outside the psychiatric clinic or hospital? Experience very quickly reveals that behavioral prescriptions work no better in the community than they do in the consulting office. On the other hand, it is equally apparent that a more active, involved stance is required of the worker in the community than is usually desirable in the treatment setting. During the period of transition—as the person new to community work is seeking to discover the nature of the role and how he can function within it—there are often periods of considerable disillusionment and even despair. The result in some cases is a retreat to the comparative safety of the clinical office (Rosenblum and Hassol, 1968). Correspondingly, there are occasional moments of deep satisfaction when a worker realizes that his sensitivity and acumen in dealing with interpersonal relations and his understanding of motivation and of mechanisms for coping with conflict allow him to help others understand and even deal more successfully with problems of adjustment in the community.

Finally, it becomes necessary to become aware of one's values and how they may influence ways of responding to the different institutions of the community and the values to be found there.

In one community, for example, a group of clergymen working with two different mental health consultants became aware that neither consultant was himself a religious person. They questioned whether they could be helped by people from other disciplines, however expert, if their values were so antithetical. As they worked with the group on this problem, it became apparent to the consultants that one of them was so biased against religion that he could not maintain sufficient objectivity and had, in fact, been raising challenging questions that represented thinly disguised attacks. The matter was discussed with the clergymen and the decision made to terminate the consultant's relationship with the group.

There are many other value and attitudinal traps into which consultants can fall, some of them far more subtle and difficult to recognize. They involve, among other possibilities, such matters as attitudes towards religious, ethnic, and national groups, political biases, and even the feelings—so pervasive in our society—that poverty is the sign of moral depravity.

I have indicated that the ultimate purpose of this book is to help the reader develop a greater appreciation of how he, in his professional role, can best fit into and contribute to the effectiveness of community life. In addition to those he has already developed as a clinical worker, what new sensitivities and skills can he bring to the community and how can they best be made available to it? To accomplish this purpose, the book encourages the worker to analyze the community in an attempt to understand its nature and dynamics, and to become as aware as possible of the forces that shape it as a habitat that supports or impairs the emotional well-being of its residents.

With an understanding of these forces, the mental health worker can become both a participant in and observer of the community in which he operates (Bruyn, 1966). He can immerse himself in a socially meaningful way in its life, while retaining the kind of detachment that fosters awareness of self and role and maintains objectivity without sacrificing commitment to the community. To do so he must have the fullest possible awareness of the limitations and potentialities of his own role in that community.

The mental health worker must avoid, for example, confusing the use of his professional role in socially meaningful ways with the civic involvement that would be appropriate if he were a citizen of the community. As a professional it is possible for him to alert the community to the probable consequences of certain decisions or courses of action; he may wish under certain circumstances to support one alternative against another. As a citizen, however, he should be freer to seek his own personal objectives along with the public good, to champion his causes, and to campaign for those he chooses. If he is perceived as using the professional role to achieve objectives in ways that are the sole prerogative of the citizen, he may jeopardize his potential effectiveness on the job.

In Wellesley a mental health consultant social worker on the staff of the agency also was a resident of the community active in civic affairs. It was possible for her to maintain a meaningful—though by no means automatic—separation between her citizen and professional stances. She was aware of the need to do so and discussed her difficulties in doing so with me and other staff members. She also made the separation explicitly for friends, neighbors, and other townspeople. The result was that colleagues trusted her with confidential information and judgments about the community; similarly, fellow townsmen trusted her with information about attitudes towards the agency and other pertinent data. The situation might have been made more difficult by the fact that she was a client of the public schools—having a child in the elementary grades—while being a consultant to school staff. Because of her own comfort and clarity about the dual roles, however, she reported no serious problems in being able to be a parent as needed on the one hand, or a consultant as required, on the other.

The important factor appears to be clarity on the part of all concerned about which hat—citizen or professional—is being worn. Here again the ability of the worker to be aware of role as well as self is essential.

DEVELOPING A SENSE OF COMMUNITY

Most of all, a *sense of community* is needed. By this is meant an awareness of the community as an entity with a pattern, a set of functions, and an identity of its own. It involves a "feel" for the ways in which the community as a habitat surrounds the individual and shapes his behavior with demands and opportunities, with constraints and freedoms, and with rewards and punishments. And it entails an appreciation of the forces which determine how decisions are made and actions taken, which in the final analysis determine whether mental health objectives are realized or not.

How does one begin the development of such a sense of community? A good way is to observe and become involved—to become both participant and observer (i.e., to use the clinical method).

In looking around the community an observer becomes aware that there are both pattern and purpose to peoples' activities there. There is a "web of community"[3] in which above all there is *movement* and it is purposeful. People are engaged in an ebb and flow of motion which varies according to the time of day and day of week, even the season of the year.

There is *concentration*. People not only live in clusters, at certain times they converge at such places as stores, schools, and churches.

There is *exchange*. Goods and services of various kinds are almost continuously being transferred from one individual or group of individuals to other individuals or groups.

There is *organization*. People belong to, participate in, owe allegiance to, are employed by, hold office in, and have responsibilities for a nearly overwhelming array of institutions, both official and unofficial. And in every community's institutions there are prescribed roles and standards of behavior which exert powerful, often irresistible demands that affect all the inhabitants in one way or another.

Perhaps most important of all, there is interpersonal interaction and *communication*. All kinds of messages are being sent and received, some of them apparently designed only to maintain human contact with a

[3] Hans Spiegel, personal communication.

minimum of friction and inconvenience, others intended to effect changes of the most far-reaching nature.

Another way is via the method of introspection. In order to enlarge his understanding of the community, an individual may begin by looking at his own community participation. How patterned are his own movements and what factors influence these movements? In what clusters does he find himself and at what times? In what sorts of exchanges of goods and services is he involved? With whom does he communicate and for what purposes? And since he is a representative of a special social movement (mental health) and its organizations, it may be of special interest to consider his participation in that movement and in the various other institutions of the community. To which does he belong? To which does he give primary allegiance? What are the roles he plays? How do these roles shape his perceptions of his own and others' behavior? How do they influence his beliefs and behavior?

Another useful way to broaden understanding of community is to make a list of all the community *roles* one plays in whatever order they come to mind. Such lists vary tremendously from person to person. Yet there are certain qualities that most lists have in common (in our society, at least). Most people place high on the list those roles that are determined by *position in the family,* such as wife or husband, son or daughter. Many go on to list their *memberships in religious and national groupings.* Almost all indicate one or more *occupational roles.* Some lists will reflect *regional and subcultural identifications, political* responsibilities, *transnational identifications,* or *special interests* and hobbies. Whatever the list, however, it quickly becomes evident that each person plays many roles in our society.

GEOGRAPHIC VERSUS FUNCTIONAL COMMUNITIES

Multiple roles are embedded within not one, and probably not two, but several communities. As noted earlier, almost everyone today relates to more than one community that is of special significance to him. There are the governmentally and geographically defined cities and towns in which we live—the collectivities that Ross (1955, 1958) has called geographic communities; and there are the other nongeographic occupational and religious groupings with which we identify and that are important to us (the entities that Ross calls functional communities).

The distinction has practical implications for the mental health team.

It is easy to confuse the two kinds of community and there is frequent danger of doing so because *in specific situations the two kinds of community often overlap*. Such confusion will usually have detrimental effects on the work being done. A case in point may help to clarify the problem.

A public health nurse-educator team wished to enlist the help of civic leaders, clergymen, and physicians in a program for the early detection and control of venereal diseases among adolescents. There was citizen interest, and local church groups, among others, gave enthusiastic support and assistance, as the health workers approached the geographic community through the board of health, local clergymen and their lay groups, and such other local organizations as the Rotary Club and League of Women Voters. The physicians of the community held back, however, until, at the suggestion of one of them, there was discussion of the proposed program with a leader of the state medical association. The statewide medical profession, through the association, constituted a significant functional community for local practitioners of medicine. Until questions about the program had been answered to the satisfaction of key people in the state medical community the local physicians could not be sure of their own position in the matter.

It should be noted in passing that the functional versus geographic distinction may come to have far less practical significance in coming decades. Geographic communities are becoming increasingly interdependent with each other, with state and national government authorities, and with a variety of professional and other functional communities. By now few decisions can be made by the local community without taking into account forces impinging on it from other jurisdictions. Thus the individual geographic community more and more becomes a member of an interlocking network of communities. These communities are bound together by regional problems and linked up with state and national units which must be called into the picture in view of the immensities of the issues to be faced. The situation increasingly resembles that of the local unit within the functional community (e.g., the local medical society *vis à vis* state and national medical associations). Functionally, therefore, the single locality becomes less independent of other localities and, indeed, becomes part of a larger regional and even federal whole.

At the very least, as is emphasized in Chapter Fifteen, the mental health worker will become increasingly involved with activities whereby the community in which he operates will need to develop effective ties with a variety of functional groups as well as with other localities and with state and federal authorities in mental health, education, and a host of other areas.

To return to the questions raised at the beginning of this chapter, what assumptions can the mental health worker make about the community? What understandings should he develop? What should "community" mean to him? The balance of the book is devoted to exploring these questions in more detail. For now I would like to make the following points:

1. It is important that the mental health worker raise the question of meaning with himself. He should ask himself from time to time what his own sense of community is and how his experiences have shaped his attitudes toward, and ability to respond to, various aspects of community life.

2. It is equally important that the worker view the community as a unified field of forces (i.e., as an interrelated and ever-shifting web wherein, to some degree or another, everything is apt to be related to all things, every action has consequences throughout the system, and all events have meaning).

3. Finally, the worker hopefully will make a major investment in community well-being which will be reflected in clearly differentiated ways in his actions as professional and citizen.

4. Just as the psychotherapist seeks to understand himself in order to understand his patients and use himself most effectively to help them cope with their problems, so the community mental health worker must seek to understand his multiple community roles and his ways of playing them out in order to understand the many facets of the community and to use himself most effectively to help groups within it cope with its many concerns.

CHAPTER THREE

Guiding Questions for the Community Mental Health Worker

Certain questions follow from the ideas discussed in the preceding chapters. The ultimate success or failure of mental health work may well depend on whether those questions are understood and whether sufficient energies are devoted both to answering them and to exploring new ones that experience is bound to uncover. To put it somewhat differently, the individual mental health worker will have the best chance of making a difference in the community when he takes nothing for granted. His questions must be basic, even naive, and often persistent. He must have the talent for creative inquiry that McNeil (1967, p. 235) has so aptly termed "a characterological distrust of the obvious."

HOW NEEDS ARE MET

I believe that the most fundamental questions for the mental health team are those having to do with how the many human needs of the population of this community are being met. The question refers to the entire hierarchy of needs from basic food and shelter to the most lofty ones of self-esteem and creativity. It has taken us too long, for example, to recognize the relative futility of such efforts as providing mental health consultation to educators working with Negro and other disadvantaged children who are convinced that even with education they are effectively barred from the job market as opposed to doing something about removing the economic barriers themselves. We must learn to ask the kinds of questions that will enable us to recognize the limitations of a program of premarital counseling in an urban setting that fails in the first place to provide sufficient opportunities for mate finding and selection.

It is important to enter the community with the recognition that one of its basic functions is to provide for the many and varied needs of its inhabitants; specialized and scarce mental health talents will be brought to bear most effectively only as we ask ourselves and the community, "Which needs are not being met and why?" The many recent experiments with special mental health services for disadvantaged groups in the inner cities have resulted from asking such questions (Riessman et al., 1964). Store front service centers manned by subprofessional workers, many of whom are drawn from the population being served, are one example of such explorations. The twenty-four hour walk-in facility at a general hospital for persons with psychosocial distress is another (Blane et al., 1967). Limited in some instances to psychiatric emergencies, the round-the-clock resource has the promise of becoming a more liberally defined helping facility that provides immediate help for less seriously distressed individuals at the times they are prepared to present themselves for help. So defined, the twenty-four hour arrangement becomes an essential component of a preventively oriented community-wide program. It facilitates case finding and early intervention; it opens up mental health services to groups that are not prepared to seek assistance on a nine-to-five basis. Such experiments are possible only because those involved take time to inquire whether existing services are the right kind to meet the needs of the populations in question.

What do we know about how help is provided in most communities to those having special needs or facing the various hazards of life? A small but growing number of inquiries into the nature of specific hazards and common patterns for help seeking is now available. The findings together with the experiences of existing mental health programs in a number of communities suggest some beginning generalizations:

1. The greatest number of mental health relevant concerns are known to clergymen, physicians, and public welfare agencies, not to mental health agencies or family service centers;

2. There are large numbers of people with problems who receive no help at all from professional sources;

3. There are a few individuals and families whose disorganization is so pervasive and chronic that they occupy a greatly disproportionate amount of uncoordinated services from a multiplicity of agencies (Buell et al., 1952);

4. The process of asking for and receiving help in our culture is both

complex and difficult. There are strong taboos against becoming dependent, and yet there are potent requirements that the individual seeking help define himself in a dependent role, such as that of patient or client, welfare recipient, or sinner, which to some extent makes him a stigmatized member of society (Goffman, 1963) ;

5. An especially promising area for collaboration between mental health teams and various community caretaking organizations is the joint investigation of ways in which supportive interventions by the caretaking groups can be strengthened to help people in times of emotional hazards.

HOW DEVIANCE IS HANDLED

Another question of significance to the mental health field is, "How is deviance handled in this community?" It is by now generally recognized that traditional treatment of major mental disorders was often based on the physical, not to mention psychological, removal of the patient from his community. There are conditions besides mental illness that tend to elicit similar patterns of rejection in many communities. Referred to here are not only the obvious groups, such as homosexuals, delinquents, or alcoholics, but also the more subtle distinctions that, in some communities, lead to marginality for those with deviant political and social views, or for such groups as teenagers who are not intellectually or culturally equipped for a college career.

Some communities exhibit better ways of handling deviance than physical removal or social isolation. They accept a wide range of political, social, and other differences. If we knew how such communities developed, it might become more possible to help all communities be more accepting and supportive of deviance when it occurs. This direction for research is especially promising and should be pursued.

HOW IDENTITIES ARE DEVELOPED

Because community mental health is dedicated to the promotion of optimal patterns of living, a third general question follows: *"How in this community are individuals enabled to develop identities that are conducive to psychological soundness and emotional well-being?"* A proper answer entails a major re-examination and basic revision of the policies, methods, and organizational patterns of the schools and other agencies responsible for the psychosocial learning of children. As Rhodes (1967) has pointed out, the basic problems of mental health and education are not to be laid at the door of education's philosophic leaders or even attributed to acknowledged skill limitations among the general run of teachers and administrators. More fundamental to our society—and expressed in many ways in every community—is a wariness of tendencies to organize and regulate the social-personal learning of individuals (Rhodes, 211). Although Rhodes concludes that such wariness results in leaving social learning to chance, I believe rather that it leaves it distributed in less explicit ways among many community institutions, not the least of which are the mass media. Exploration of this question in any community would entail familiarity with its various socializing agencies, including not only the family and the schools, but also the churches, youth agencies, voluntary associations serving those having special needs, adult education and county extension programs, and agencies and organizations serving the elderly, to name only a few. An answer also entails an assessment of those not well-served by such agencies, whose encounters with the community leave them stigmatized and psychologically impaired.

The remainder of this book does not deal directly with such issues as treatment and prevention. Instead it is concerned with questions of a different kind, having to do with problems and processes with which anyone who seeks to change community patterns in order to achieve the focal objectives of mental health is involved: the development of communities wherein help is available when needed, and healthy psychological development is promoted. The questions to be raised in this regard, it seems to me, arise from a commitment to influence the quality of community life in significant ways, and to seek social change when it seems indicated. The mental health worker is inevitably an agent of change. As such, it is important for him to go about his business with the fullest possible awareness of what he is doing and of the kinds of dynamics with which he is dealing.

In any particular community it is important to try to discover how decisions are made and who makes them. Section 2 contains a conceptualization of elements and processes that hopefully will orient the reader toward the various forces that operate to affect the quality and nature of decisions within the complex social system that is the community.

A word of caution is in order, however. Traditionally trained mental health workers will find it difficult to develop a comfortable stance as change agents. They will frequently re-experience what a colleague [4] describes as "the terrible awkwardness" they felt when, as budding psychotherapists, they tried on for size various new intrapsychic and interpersonal knowledge. There are two dangers. On the one hand, the individ-

[4] Dr. S. Eugene Long, NIMH

ual may retreat from the new awkwardness to become nothing but a clinician after all. On the other hand, he may tend to foreswear his unique focus on individual psychology in favor of challenging new social reform possibilities. Either way he loses the opportunity to develop a broader mental health identity rooted in his original core of clinical skills and sophistication. It is virtually essential that as he goes through the new period of terrible awkwardness the individual has the support of a reference group of colleagues with whom he can hammer out problems and share both uncertainties and enthusiasms. It is also helpful if individuals retain at least a part-time investment in clinical work or its equivalent with individuals or groups.

Fact finding and inquiry are essential functions for the agent of change. Research, when properly used, becomes a powerful resource that can be used to illuminate new prospects and possibilities for improved mental health. It is important, therefore, that we ask ourselves, "How can inquiry be so conducted in this community that its results can be accepted and used most effectively?" Section 3 is devoted to a consideration of this question.

There is a whole series of questions to be raised in connection with change itself. How does change typically come about in this community? To what extent is the community oriented to accept change? What factors will determine whether a particular innovation will be accepted or rejected? Closely related to such questions are queries related to conflict: To what kinds of conflict is the community susceptible? How do conflicts arise? Having arisen, how are they managed? To what extent does the community's ways of handling conflicts tend to resolve them? Section 4 treats the community as a place where differing interests, values, and viewpoints meet and often clash; where mental health values must contend with other, sometimes conflicting, approaches; and where disagreements must in some way be dealt with. There is one chapter devoted entirely to the question of how, despite cleavage and conflict, communities manage to maintain both some degree of internal integration and external ties with groups and forces on the outside.

Finally, there is the matter of moving within a community in a planned, organized way toward the solution of problems and the accomplishment of predetermined goals. What are this community's patterns for problem solving? Under what circumstances, and in what ways, will its citizens mobilize for action? How effectively does the community act to achieve specific objectives? These questions are explored in Section 5, which seeks to present a conceptual framework that can be used to plan and evaluate the steps needed to mobilize community groups for change.

2

Theoretical Perspectives on Community

"There are many dimensions in this new planning for community-based mental health services. The community is as real as the house next door and as ethereal as poetic feelings of kinship with groups of people anywhere on earth. The problem we face involves not only new techniques of administering a program supported by federal, state, local, and private funds. We must also maintain a deep concern with each individual as we concurrently become concerned with the welfare of all the people."

BERTRAM S. BROWN, M.D., *Deputy Director, National Institute of Mental Health*

(1967, p. 5)

CHAPTER FOUR

The Community as a Social System

OVERVIEW

How are decisions made in any community? Who determines how the myriad of agencies, institutions, and informal groupings with their rules, laws, codes, and customs, impinge on the individual for his ultimate good or ill-being?

On first consideration we face a complex and even chaotic state of affairs. Many decisions, for example, are made at the level of personal choice; others involve the more or less deliberate acts of groups. Some pertain to matters falling exclusively within the purview of the group or organization which makes the decision. Other decisions, such as attempts to invoke censorship of books and films, affect many people such as children, who have little or nothing to say about them. Some decisions are made as a choice between clear alternatives. Some have far-reaching effects, sometimes neither understood nor anticipated by those making them. Some decisions are publicly arrived at; others are made outside the range of public scrutiny. Some are definite acts of a deliberate nature; others represent decisions by default or even neglect. There are managed decisions; decisions left to the natural interplay of forces; or decisions based on struggle and contention. There are decisions arrived at through the coercive imposition of force, through negotiation, or through consensus.

All of these kinds of decisions occur in any single community in the course of a short period of time. Yet the result somehow is not chaos, but patterning. The patterning represents a kind of interplay of formal and informal structures and their functioning, which, in most communities at any rate, are remarkably responsive to the needs of large numbers of their inhabitants.

A colleague [5] is fond of posing the question, "If you had the responsibility for feeding people, how would you plan to arrange things in a metropolitan area of several million people so that everyone would be fed approximately three times a day and would eat just about the kind of food he prefers and, with few exceptions, would receive sufficient quantities to maintain life and health?" The task staggers the imagination. It requires careful consideration of food-growing capabilities; transportation, storage, and distribution facilities; awareness of food preferences on the part of millions of people from differing sociocultural backgrounds; problems of food preparation; recruitment and training of food handlers; maintenance of supplies of dishes, linen, packaging materials, and so on. Yet somehow, despite inefficiencies and considerable inequities, every major community in this country manages without centralized planning to deal with the problem. How can we account for processes whereby the food problem is "solved" not once but repeatedly, day after day, year after year in such communities despite shifts in climate and eating habits? The beginnings of an answer appear to lie in the concept of community as a social system. This concept suggests that the community is a more or less integrated and self-correcting arrangement of structures and processes which are able to transmit, process, interpret, and act on great amounts of information. Such a social system view is not easy to grasp. It is abstract because it attempts to account for interrelationships among the fantastically complex array of actors and events which make up community life. To the extent that it is successful, however, it can be an effective aid to the mental health worker as he plans programs, maps strategies, and assesses day-to-day activities.

FOUR BASIC PROCESSES

The concept emphasizes patterned interaction of certain key elements, including goals, norms, and roles (Moe, 1959). In attempting to grasp the concept it helps to recognize that we are used to thinking similarly of individual personality. It is possible, for example, to substitute community goals for individuals' needs or motives, community norms for individuals' attitudes and values, and community roles for individuals' character structure.

In thinking about the community, therefore, the shift is made to transindividual elements. Groups and organizations have goals; norms to some degree guide the conduct of all those having membership in a col-

[5] Professor John Glidewell, University of Chicago.

lectivity, no matter what their personal predilections; and roles refer to the patterning of behavior which results from generally agreed on expectations of those who occupy certain positions within the society.

In practice, for example in negotiating a mental health program with a superintendent of schools, it is at least as important to be familiar with the role of the superintendent in modern American communities (Gross et al., 1958) as to be aware of the particular superintendent's personality and characteristic ways of coping. For it is the *role* of the superintendent, the *norms* of his functional community of educators, and the *goals* of the education program that will determine, far more than will his personality, the ways in which he can respond to the mental health field.

Community system theorists such as Loomis (1960) and Moe (1959) have identified certain processes which they consider essential to the interplay of such elements as goals, norms, and roles. To quote Moe (p. 27), "The particular content of the elements and the nature of the processes in turn give a certain uniqueness of character to the community."

We shall consider four types of processes: (a) communication, (b) decision making, (c) systemic linkage (the linking that takes place between systems or between the several subsystems involved in a complex system), and (d) boundary maintenance (the activity which has the function of preserving and strengthening the system itself). All four are involved simultaneously in the successful accomplishment of any community function (C. F. Jonassen, 1959). Nevertheless, for purposes of clarity each is discussed separately as though it functions independently.

COMMUNICATION

Community cannot exist without communication. Its communication patterns are the means whereby all other aspects are maintained and expressed. Without channels for communication, there could be no interplay between populations and their habitats, no impact of past history on current beliefs, no carrying out of community functions; in short, no community.

Communication patterns reflect all other aspects of the community in much the same way that the reading of a thermometer reflects the functioning of bodily processes. Difficulties in communication often are symptomatic of other problems or concerns. Moreover, solutions of such problems often must include alteration of communication channels and of the nature of the communication. One anthropologist, Chapple

(1955), asserts that interpersonal and intergroup problems within organizations can be resolved by analysis and alteration of interaction patterns alone *without regard to the contents of such interactions.* Whether or not one accepts such total de-emphasis of content, there is little doubt that communication patterns do tend to reflect as well as affect other organizational and community characteristics. For instance, regardless of the content of the exchanges, a community in which citizens in the mental health association are in frequent contact with school board members will probably have a far different educational mental health program than one in which the two groups have little or no contact.

Communication is not only the act by which information is exchanged; neither is it only the information which is being exchanged. More adequate for understanding community events is the view held by information theorists that communication is *purposive;* that is, it occurs when an individual or group seeks to influence (in other words, to change) another individual or group. It is in the reception of ideas and their translation into behavior that communication truly occurs. As Ruesch and Bateson (1951, p. 6) put it, "all actions and events have communicative aspects, as soon as they are perceived by a human being; [such a definition] implies, furthermore, that such perception changes the information which an individual possesses and therefore influences him."

By the same token, individuals are influenced by what is *not* transmitted or is transmitted in a fragmentary way. Any psychotherapist knows that the achievement of adequate communication can be and often is a tremendously complex and difficult task. The problem of ensuring agreement about the meanings of words is difficult enough. But that is only the beginning. Communication is more than content. It also involves the attitudes of the communicator (to content, to self, and to receiver), not to mention the receiver's perception of these attitudes. There are also the intentions toward one another of those involved in the communication process, which must be taken into account. Even in relatively simple face-to-face communications between persons who share a common task or have some other bond (e.g., psychotherapy) the parties often have difficulty knowing and understanding one another's meanings, attitudes, or intentions. An underlying issue in the mental health worker's attempts to communicate with people in the community is that of whether he will open himself up to others' influence when he is simultaneously seeking to influence them. Psychotherapy, in the classic sense at least, tends to place the therapist outside the influence of the patient. Communication in the community must be more reciprocal.

The mental health worker in the community is faced with an infinitely more difficult set of problems than he faced in his office because the situations are apt to be more complex, working arrangements less clear, and contacts more fleeting and superficial. Let us consider an example from a community case in a field other than mental health.

It was possible recently to observe the interplay of factors affecting communication and ultimate decision making about fluoridation in a small upper-middle-class community. The town meeting members, many of them well-educated and scientifically sophisticated, rejected fluoridation of the water supply by a sizable margin, despite the strong recommendations of the health officer. The latter, a respected and well known person, had briefly and clearly presented the facts regarding the safety and effectiveness of fluorides. Interviews with a few town meeting members, all college graduates, revealed some interesting data which have relevance to communication. One respondent said, for example, "There were not enough facts; how much of a health problem is it?"

The case reflects the fact that selection of content to be communicated in a community situation often is made—sometimes necessarily so—on the basis of inadequate knowledge of what information is needed or wanted.

A number of studies have indicated that communication is fragmented and inefficient, and often leads to serious distortions and misunderstandings, when emotions or cherished beliefs are involved. Griffiths and Knutson (1960, p. 521), reviewing such studies and their implications for public health workers, comment: "The evidence suggests that achieving long-term attitude and behavior change requires communications of a more personal type to assure full understanding of the meaning of the change and to help in translating the change into the personal behavior of the individual concerned." An illustration of their point occurs in the fluoridation case.

Another respondent reported, "I voted to support the minority, who seemed so genuinely upset about being forced to drink something they feared." There seemed to be three aspects of this response. First, as in the previous case, the individual had not been given necessary facts about the urgency of the health problem; second, she acted on a value position, which places minority rights above health considerations; third, she seemed to imply a callous attitude toward the opponents on the part of the health experts and their supporters. This respondent did not perceive any commonality or sense of shared community participation between the health group and the opponents of fluoridation. She may have been expressing a greater degree of identification with an aroused fellow citizen than with a professional health authority, whom she may have perceived as being more interested in scientific fact than in citizen feeling.

Many problems arise from the fact that in one community situation after another, individuals and groups attempt to communicate to those with whom they do not, and perhaps cannot, identify. The signal for such absence of identification is often the appearance of "me-you" or "we-they" language, which implies a feeling of apartness and essential

difference in worth between those involved. Far too frequently such social distance results in the formation and reinforcement of stereotypes,
wherein the assumptions made about others' motivations are not the
same as those made about one's own. Such concerns about motivation
were raised in the fluoridation case.

A third respondent raised a question about the intentions of the pro-fluoridation
group. He said, "Frankly, I couldn't help wondering why the health officer was in
such a rush to push this thing across." In the current fluoridation controversies
around the nation each side views the other with suspicion, mistrust, and hostility.
Antifluoridationists are perceived as crackpots who are trying to turn the clock
back on science and progress; profluoridationists are perceived as communists or the
tools of big business interests. The intentions of both sides are perceived by their
antagonists in the most malevolent ways. As a consequence, each side tends to be
completely suspicious of any act or attempt to communicate on the part of the
other.

Communication Channels. As has been indicated already, networks
of communication channels exist in every community which tend to direct the flow of information and the attempts at influence along more or
less regularly used pipelines. Some individuals and groups have greater
access to and influence within such channels than do others. It is also
true that multiple networks of communication channels exist in every
community. Most information tends to flow more freely within certain
networks than others. Similarly, most individuals are located within certain networks and are denied access to others. Attempts at communication of mental health messages, therefore, must take into account the
probability that no single effort to communicate with a large segment of
the people in any community will be successful. Efforts to communicate
widely must be carried out through those individuals and media which
have access to the greatest number of relevant communication nets. The
importance of locating the most relevant network is exemplified in the
following case.

In a community of approximately 20,000 people a small group was interested in
re-establishing an annual Fourth of July celebration which before World War II
had been a highly successful tradition. The group, composed primarily of newcomers, was not successful in its efforts until it enlisted the enthusiastic support of
the owner of a small neighborhood grocery store in a section inhabited primarily
by the "old families" of the town. The grocer was a native. Though not a high-
status figure or a person with any power in the community, his work brought him
into contact with hundreds of the old residents. Moreover, he was a jovial, garru-
lous person who loved to gossip and was known as one who had the best interests
of the town at heart. Very quickly almost everyone in the community knew that
there was going to be a July 4 celebration. The grocer became the focal point for
committees working on the program, decorations, the parade, refreshments, fire-
works, and the like. The original group watched in amazement as scores of people

became involved, public interest mounted, the newspapers swung behind the project, and merchants hastened to donate prizes. Everyone said later that the grocer had done a great job for the town in thinking up and spark-plugging the renewal of the tradition.

Mass Media. The task of communication is often simplified when newspapers, radio, and television are available. Even such media, however, offer no panacea. There are those in any community who neither look at nor listen to them. They are limited, too, by restrictions of space or time, and by their one-way nature, which under some conditions impedes accuracy of understanding.

As Griffiths and Knutson (1960) have pointed out, communication by newspaper, radio, or television can be effective in conveying factual information or even in altering attitudes, but is relatively ineffective when the issues involved are highly controversial and emotionally charged. Mass media also may generate and maintain cohesiveness in the community, therefore helping to maintain effective citizen participation in meeting community problems.

When I was involved in a community development program in a New England village, I noticed increased civic pride and cohesiveness on the part of citizens when the regional newspaper was persuaded by merchants and other town leaders to include in each issue a separate two-page section devoted to village matters.

Factors Affecting Access to Communications. Many factors affect access to communication channels. Among them are physical proximity and socioeconomic status.

Physical proximity: Amount and accuracy of communication may be affected by as simple a factor as propinquity. Studies of housing developments, for example, have shown that one is far more likely to interact with the next door neighbor than with a person three houses down on a corner lot. There are places in any community where people congregate regularly, such as the laundromat, the shopping center, the corner meat market, the town dump, or the neighborhood bar. Such places serve as significant communication centers and those who spend time there will usually have access to far more information than those who do not.

Socioeconomic status: A person's role and status in the community will also influence his position within its communication networks. Officials are aware of certain channels from which others are excluded. Organizational memberships also play a part, since exchange of information within groups is usually more open than communication between groups. Members of more favored social groups are also apt to have been educated better than disadvantaged individuals in the matter of knowing how to locate and use the spectrum of available channels.

Formal and Informal Communication: Communication nets within communities include both formal, official, and publicly recognized channels and a great variety of informal, unofficial pipelines. Both types have been studied extensively within organizations. Among other things, we know that formal channels in most effective organizations exist between those whose roles are complementary. There are also formally defined channels between functionally related persons of unequal status, such that each person in a hierarchy knows to whom he must report and, conversely, to whom he must transmit information of a directing or controlling nature.

Both formal and informal channels are essential if adequate communication is to take place. It is true that individuals do sometimes deplore the existence of irresponsible "rumor mongers." The complicated nature of the community, however, as well as the continuously shifting problems to be dealt with, suggest that at worst informal channels are inevitable and that at best, they are necessary if effective adaptation to new concerns and circumstances is to occur.

Studies of rumors in communities and institutions such as mental hospitals, have highlighted the potency of such channels. They have revealed that informal means are utilized with great rapidity when formal networks have broken down, or when for any reason they are unavailable. In and of themselves, informal channels are neither good nor bad. On the one hand, they may add variety and adaptability to efforts at dealing with problems. Sometimes, for example, it is possible by means of informal contacts to arrive at solutions in situations which might become locked in irreconcilable open conflict if formal channels alone are utilized. Much community decision making and problem solving goes on informally with formal meetings of boards and committees serving simply to record and legalize decisions. Indeed, formal and informal exchanges in most well functioning community situations usually are complementary and can be viewed as parts of a well integrated whole.

On the other hand, there are times when informal communication becomes dysfunctional. Open meetings of public boards and councils often are necessary lest those not "in the know" develop distrust of officials' motives or lest those in power fail to recognize or take into account the legitimate concerns of those affected by their deliberations. When informal communications become destructive and serve only to increase hostilities and anxieties, existing formal or official communication networks may need to be overhauled or new ones developed in order to include otherwise alienated individuals and groups.

Various methods have been tried for the development of more effective and inclusive means for communication and community problem solving. Among them are *ad hoc* citizen action groups based on informal networks among those not holding official positions or formal roles (Alinsky, 1946), neighborhood or block associations as formal organizations bringing together people of diverse backgrounds at the local level (Thelen, 1954), and the more prevalent councils of lay people or professionals representing the health and social agencies of a community. Each has proved successful in some cases and for certain purposes. With the growing need for massive community planning efforts, in which problems of physical and social planning must be faced together, increasing attention will no doubt be given to the systematic development and use of communication channels (such as the use of electronic means for rapidly registering public opinion) to facilitate citizen participation in the affairs of ever more complex communities. Indeed, such deliberate, planned use of communication will become increasingly necessary simply as a means of enabling citizens to function effectively in the complex, large, rapidly changing communities of which they are a part.

MAINTENANCE OF BOUNDARIES

"Every five years city and town officials must walk the bounds of their community. Last week, the Wayland selectmen teamed up with a representative of the Natick Board of Selectmen to perambulate, find, and mark the bounds between the two towns." [6]

This quaint and archaic custom is believed to have its origins in mediaeval church procedure in England when church officials regularly surveyed parish property. The parish later became a political instrument and the custom of perambulation was brought by religious groups to colonial communities in the new world. Even in the early colonial days, procedures were needed to ensure that intercommunity territorial boundaries could be established and maintained.

Boundary maintenance problems are both geographic and social. They are not the kind which can be settled by any simple custom such as boundary perambulation. They are brought about by such things as the rapid inflex of large groups of newcomers and by urban sprawl. Also, most of us exist psychologically within multiple communities, each with its own distinct areas and jurisdiction. For the suburban commuter, his work community may be the central city, and the bedroom community the suburb; the shopping community may embrace two or more towns served by a gigantic shopping plaza; the school jurisdiction may be consolidated with still other towns or areas within a county, and

[6] *The Town Crier*, Wayland, Mass., December 16, 1965, p. 43.

so on. Under such circumstances it is sometimes difficult to determine which groups should be committed to any particular community effort such as mental health. Uncertainty also arises about the extent to which such seeming outsiders as mental health professionals are or should be identified with "our town." Boundaries are as much social as they are physical in nature.

Boundary maintenance thus is complicated by the fact that boundaries are topographic, politicosociologic, and sociopsychologic in nature. Whatever its characteristics, any boundary has the function of regulating the passage of people or ideas between or within regions. Communities vary greatly in the nature of their boundary maintenance. Some are far more receptive to strangers and new ideas (e.g., mental health ideas that are readily received in an upper-middle-class suburb may be less welcome in an urban ethnic ghetto). Particular kinds of newcomers such as psychiatrists will be more readily received in one community than in others. It is clear that much can be learned about any community by a study of how the input of new people and ideas is regulated at its boundary.

Community boundary maintenance is not readily visible to the casual observer. To those most directly affected, however, it is often palpable indeed. Ethnic or racial groups unable to move into certain communities can testify to the existence of boundaries which for them serve as barriers to in-migration. Boundaries exist, however, even when they do not serve to exclude. There is always some resistance to passage through a boundary, though it may not be experienced as such. Passage, as the word is used here, may or may not be physical movement through space. It is always a psychological phenomenon. It involves the attitudes, feelings, and identifications of the individual as well as significant roles and relationships. Physical phenomena often create or reinforce the boundaries of which we speak, and psychological movement across them is frequently facilitated or impeded by major physical changes.

The construction of a large, new superhighway through a village on the outskirts of a major city resulted in an increased rate of population expansion and division of the town into two discrete sections north and south of the artery. At the next town meeting, residents experienced their first major controversy over the location of a new elementary school. Until then all schools had been placed in the center of the village on a common site. Now many believed the community should shift to a neighborhood-school concept. Older residents, believing that the community should continue to be one homogeneous "neighborhood," opposed the change. They argued that neighborhood schools would create artificial barriers between social groups. The town became split politically as a result of the new physical boundary and the increased rate of influx of newcomers.

DECISION MAKING AND POWER

Untold numbers of decisions are made in the typical community, even the smallest town, in the course of one year. The web of such decision making is extremely complex, and yet each community appears to have its unique style of identifying salient issues or concerns and arriving at decisions about them. In one community, for example, significant decisions may be made quietly and unobtrusively by a tightly knit top group of leaders; in another, no decision of any moment is made without bitter and open conflict between traditionally warring factions. Of special interest to the mental health field is Freeman's (1960) discovery that the same community circles, leaders, and organizations were not involved in such apparently similar matters as mental health, and such public health concerns as the establishment of a new hospital or medical school. Moreover, the health leaders for the most part were not overtly linked to the leadership involved in city planning and economic development programs.

There are some clear implications for mental health workers in the conclusion that communities vary tremendously in the extent to which leadership is concentrated or is spread widely among a range of business and civic organizations. Obviously the problem of developing and implementing a community program in mental health will be quite different in a community governed by a cohesive, strong, single top leadership group than in a community in which a number of more or less independent and even conflicting factions all participate in the influence structure. It is apparent that we would be well advised to use whatever means we can to determine the nature and distribution of the top leadership structure in each community in which a mental health program is located.

In making such an assessment we must be careful to search out the informal and less apparent influentials who may affect certain kinds of decisions. Informal decision makers operating within informal structures may be even more potent at times than the more formal recognized leaders (Ross, 1955).

INFLUENCE AND COMMUNITY LEADERSHIP

There is a valuable and growing body of literature among political scientists about the nature and quality of community decision making.

Much of it was stimulated by Hunter's classic study of Atlanta, Georgia (Hunter, 1953) which, using a reputational method for identifying community leaders, came forth with the suggestion that community policies were established by a small group of top elite business, investment, and political figures with a professional person or two thrown in for good measure.

The rash of studies following Hunter's work have tended to modify Hunter's thesis. Communities appear to vary in the extent to which influence is concentrated in the hands of an elite group or distributed among two or more blocs. One of the most carefully documented studies was made in Syracuse, New York (Freeman, 1960, 1962). It revealed that several different leadership and organizational clusters were involved in the solution of community problems. Moreover, different types of problems attracted quite different leadership clusters. Freeman and his associates identified three kinds of community leaders:

1. The *influentials* appear to be very similar to Hunter's group of top policy makers. They are the heads of large banks and corporations as well as a few political leaders whose organizations play a part in major community projects.

2. The *effectors* represent top management and technical specialists who operate more directly with specific community projects under the auspices of the influentials and their organizations.

3. The *activists* are the leaders of voluntary organizations and associations who play prominent roles in certain community issues (among them, presumably, would be mental health), but tend not to be represented in others involving major economic decisions.

When it comes to the implementation of health plans, there is some evidence to support the common-sense notion that when permanent leadership of the community is involved (i.e., citizens who remain in the locality) as against temporary leadership (i.e., the typically more mobile professional health leaders), there is more chance for follow-through. (James and Mico, 1964) It is an unfortunate fact that professionals in some community fields, among them mental health, do not stay long enough to form the informal associations upon which change can be based. Decisions informally arrived at by those not apparently involved may have far-reaching significance for community problem solving behavior, acceptance of change and the like, especially when the formal and informal structures happen not to be aligned with reference to any particular issue. An example cited by Ross was an unsuccessful attempt to introduce a new type of seed into an agricultural community through educational approaches to the men, who as farmers were part of the formal agricultural structure. Effective resistance to the new seed came from the women, part of the informal "housewife-consumer" structure, who objected to the quality of the flour produced.

SOCIAL VERSUS RATIONAL-TECHNICAL APPROACHES TO DECISIONS

One of the challenges of decision making in today's society is that of providing the means whereby the information, viewpoints, and awareness of needs which can come only from the local level are combined with the broad perspective, technical skill, and scientific knowledge possessed by authorities at the regional, national, and international levels. The difficulties of arriving at such a synthesis are well illustrated by the problems encountered in recent years when technically competent city planners and architects have sought to enter into effective problem solving relationships with neighborhood groups.

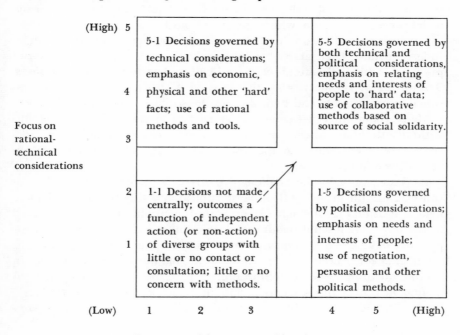

Focus on social process considerations

Figure 1. Two-dimensional framework for analysis of decision making: rational-technical and social process (R.A.S.P.). General time phases in the decision making sequence: (a) Awareness of a problem or issue; (b) Becoming familiar with the problem, data gathering and defining the problem; (c) Considering alternatives; (d) Deciding a course of action; (e) Effecting and implementing the course of action.

At a conference on decision making in complex metropolitan areas (Franklin and Franklin, 1967), I participated in the development of a two-dimensional scheme for the analysis of the interplay between technical and social psychological factors in arriving at community decisions. The scheme presented in Figure 1 assumes that all decisions are arrived at through varying admixtures of concern with rational or technical techniques and considerations on the one hand, and with social processes such as the attitudes, needs biases, political maneuvers, value clashes, and other considerations arising out of the psychological nature of those involved, on the other hand. Any decision can be rated according to whether it is judged to have been arrived at through rational-technical or social means, or both.

A decision located at the upper left-hand quadrant of Figure 1 is judged to have been arrived at primarily through rational and technical means. Social processes were not taken into account. We give this kind of decision a rating of 5-1 to indicate that the decision was high (5) on the rational-technical scale, which runs from 1 to 5, and low (1) on the social process dimension, which also runs from 1 to 5.

Conversely, a decision located at the lower right-hand quadrant is judged to have been arrived at primarily through concern with social processes, with little attention to rational and technical considerations. The rating of 1-5 means that the decision is scored low (1) on the rational-technical scale and high (5) on the social process dimension.

Many community decisions are arrived at more or less by default, without attention either to rational or social considerations. Such a decision would be located at the lower left quadrant and is low (1) on both dimensions.

If as suggested in the challenge referred to earlier, local needs and concerns are integrated with broad technical and scientific skills of planners, a decision may be high (5) on both dimensions and thus be located in the upper right-hand quadrant.[7] Community decisions in my own experience have fallen at various points in the diagram. I find that there is a tendency for decisions in certain areas of community life to fall within similar quadrants and to follow similar patterns. The development of mental health facilities seems to fall into such a pattern. In the early days the decision to establish a mental health association or begin work

[7] A similar two-dimensional framework for analysis of organizational patterns has been developed by Robert Blake. It is described in the book *The Managerial Grid* (Blake and Mouton, Gulf Publishing, Houston, Texas, 1964). Blake's dimensions juxtapose concern for or emphasis on task (i.e., organizational production) and person. The present scheme for analysis of community decisions was stimulated by Blake's analytical approach.

toward the development of a clinic often is 1-5 (i.e., based largely on social processes and the personal concerns of those involved). Later, however, after clinics have been established, decisions on policies and practices are 5-1; they are for the most part decided by clinic staff and are made largely on the basis of best available scientific knowledge and professional standards. In communities where no individuals have risen to the challenge, a "decision" not to develop a mental health facility is usually made by default (1-1 in Figure 1). Some of the recent comprehensive approaches to statewide planning for mental health have done an outstanding job of integrating the technical judgments of professional leaders from many different disciplines with the values, concerns, and felt needs of citizens.

Decisions, Leadership Style, and Type of Organization. The personal styles or organizational leaders no doubt influence how their organizations go about making decisions. A free-wheeling individual with high autonomy needs is not likely to run a tight, procedurally obsessed bureaucracy. Similarly, a person who values system and order is not likely to manage an organization that is readily responsive to new and novel inputs. Warren (1967) proposes a rough three-part typology of organizational leadership styles: "charismatic," "bureaucratic," and "collegial." The charismatic leader emphasizes personal innovation and an *ad hoc* approach to problems and projects. The bureaucratic leader, much as in the popular stereotype of "The Bureaucrat," plays the organizational game according to an established rulebook of policies, precedents, guidelines, and hierarchical procedural channels. Collegial leadership combines the elements of flexibility in decision making procedures and emphasis on involvement of subordinates in decisions wherever feasible, no matter where they may be on the administrative ladder.

Warren suggests that certain organizational structures and missions encourage particular leadership styles and decisional approaches. My own experiences confirm this hypothesis. It is probably not accidental that welfare departments so often have bureaucratically inclined individuals in responsible positions. It is no more accidental that the "war on poverty" has been headed by a person willing, able, and inclined to improvise in the best charismatic style. And in those established organizations requiring the effective synthesis of diverse viewpoints and talents in order to achieve success (e.g., modern organizations and community councils) leadership is predictably collegial more often than chance would allow.

One of the differences between traditional mental institutions and the modern community based agency lies in their decisional styles. Bureaucratic decision making is maladaptive in situations requiring new responses to new conditions, such as those faced by community mental health centers. It is also hard to imagine a successful mental health center flourishing over the long pull under charismatic leadership conditions. The very multidisciplinary nature of the community mental health task requires the fullest use of the diverse skills of a variegated staff. Under the circumstances I predict that collegially inclined leaders will have the best chance to succeed and survive.

Decisions at Different Phases of Community Action. Studies of community action programs indicate that the quality and nature of decision making vary according to the phase of action in which a project finds itself. Initiators of community action may be helped to decide whether or not to launch a project by consultation with friends, neighbors, business associates, or persons believed to have the community's interests at heart. Somewhat later, an informal group may be formed to explore the problem further and to decide whether to move into a phase of formal and public action. Finally, more formal auspices for action must be established and a program launched. How decisions are made at any phase will depend to some extent on who is involved and on an assessment of what next steps must be taken. Questions must be considered, such as, "Under whose auspices should the project be conducted?" "Should there be a wide appeal for citizen support?" "Should the strategy be limited to approaching only those involved in the final decision making body?" These questions are taken up more thoroughly in Section 5.

Decisions at Times of Crisis. In crisis situations otherwise quiescent individuals and groups tend to shift rapidly into action. At such times people become impatient with deliberate approaches to problem appraisal and decision making. Hostility arises, tension increases, and action becomes impulsive. Alternatives are rarely examined. It is also interesting to note that support is usually quickly mobilized behind anyone who presents a clear, simple, direct solution or plan of action. A Red Cross official at a talk I heard some years ago described how such leadership developed during the Cameron Parish Flood disaster in Louisiana:

> When regular government services broke down and Red Cross crews moved in to help citizens deal with the crisis, a relatively uneducated, previously unknown carpenter emerged as someone who took action, looked out for others, and could be relied on to bring people together when the Red Cross team needed them.

Similar leadership emergence has been reported by other disaster teams. Usually such leaders do not maintain leadership after the crisis has subsided.

Under crisis conditions, thoughtful community decision making is rarely achieved. Simple action steps are sought and considerable pressure is often brought to bear in efforts to seek solutions. In the process certain individuals or groups may find themselves singled out for attack.

A suburban community was faced with a crisis involving a series of tragic automobile accidents in which a number of adolescents were killed and injured. One of the accidents was an apparent suicide. When it became known that one teen-age driver had been drinking, groups sprang up demanding that officials take action to raise the minimum driver age and crack down on teen-age drinking. At a well attended meeting townspeople became incensed when one official contended that serious automobile accidents involving adolescents were not unduly frequent in the younger age group, so that raising the minimum age would not ameliorate the situation. The mental health agency sent an observer to the meeting but found in informal conversations that it was not possible at the time to direct attention to broader and more basic concerns having to do with the needs of adolescents in the community.

Once the crisis conditions have abated, it is usually possible for those involved to examine remaining problems in greater depth and to consider actions which might forestall future problems of a similar kind. This was the case in the suburban community facing unmet needs of adolescents.

Contest Strategies for Decisions. It is taken for granted in a democracy that many, if not most, decisions (especially those involving government) should be made on a majority basis in response to a yes-no definition of the problem. When the choice is between competing values, there is probably no better way of deciding. Yet I believe that an over-commitment to this decision making pattern has unfavorable effects. One concomitant of the method is that most people become involved in community decision making or are mobilized for action only at the time of the final acceptance or rejection of a particular alternative, or when —as in the case of election to office—a choice must be made between two or possibly three competing candidates.

Studies of the decision making process in relation to such things as adequacy, rapidity, and implementation of decisions indicate that the yes-no approach has serious limitations for community problem solving. First, it tends to polarize the community into fixed and often warring factors; second, it creates a win-lose situation in which the losers (who may be as many as 49% of those involved) may feel that the decision was not a sound one; third, it discourages the examination of all possible alternatives and the creative discovery of new solutions; fourth, it heightens the possibility that large segments of the population will have little commitment either to the decision or to the steps which are needed to implement it.

It is apparent, however, that the American political system, predicated on a contest model, has worked reasonably well. It has solved problems, created civic commitment, permitted decisions, and allowed for change; marred as it may be at times by corruption and alienation of certain segments of the population. Perhaps the system works so well just because tradeoffs and accommodations occur, as Long[8] puts it, "behind and around the yes-no decisions."

Consensus in Community Decisions. In recent years increased attention has been paid to the method of consensus in decision making, partly through the example set by the Quakers and partly because research in the small group field has indicated that, when feasible, the method is highly effective. In this method the commitment of group members is to arrive at a decision that represents a synthesis of the needs and points of view of as many members as possible. Action is deferred until all concerned agree with or at least assent to it. The consensus method is not an easy one to adopt, especially for people inured to yes-no, win-lose decision making. It is feasible, however, especially where there is a genuine commitment to one another on the part of all group members, coupled with a sense of mutual respect and trust.

Its use also helps create the conditions in which trust and community solidarity can emerge. I believe, therefore, that the consensus approach warrants wider use than it now enjoys. It is also clear that no single approach to decision making is the best under all circumstances, either in terms of the quality of the decision itself or of the welfare of the community as a whole.

Conflict Strategies. In recent years we have witnessed the emergence of civil disobedience strategies and so-called conflict strategies whereby one group mobilizes moral force, economic sanctions, and other means to gain its objectives against hard-core opposition (Alinsky, 1946; Poston, 1953). These practices, too, have worked when consensus was impossible and traditional contest methods had been impotent for decades. Yet in the long run severe and protracted community conflict can leave serious scars of antagonism and mistrust.

Mental health workers, if they are sensitive to the range of available decision making approaches, may be able to facilitate the use of those that will encourage community cohesiveness and increased trust among groups.

Understanding of Power. Social power can be considered equivalent to energy or force, or, more strictly speaking, a combination of forces

8 Dr. S. Eugene Long, personal communication.

that can bring about, sustain, or, for that matter, prevent, change (Clark, 1966). To understand power, however, we must understand its sources, how it is perceived, and how it is used by those engaged in political, social, or economic change.

An understanding of the multiple sources, locations, and expressions of power in the community is fundamental to our understanding of decision making. Power is always being exerted, through legitimate authority or in less formalized ways, in order to ensure the performance of necessary community functions. We must confront power realistically and discard commonly held simplistic notions of power in favor of a more differentiated concept.

From a common sense point of view, power involves the use of superior forces of one sort or another to accomplish one's ends. A more sophisticated definition views power as *the ability of an individual or a group to realize its will in a communal action despite resistance from others participating in the situation* (Weber, 1946). This view emphasizes that the ability to influence stems from any one of a number of sources. Thus the proverbial "power of an idea" may refer to any one of several possibilities: (a) the idea may be expressed persuasively (i.e., powerfully), (b) the individual expressing it may enhance the idea with the power of his own prestige, status, or authority, (c) those presenting the idea may have the power to exert command over many media for its dissemination, or (d) as in the original meaning of the phrase, the idea may derive great power from its essential appropriateness to the problem at hand. Power then becomes *the ability to command those resources relevant to the needs of the individuals and groups most concerned in any specific context.*

Power is multidimensional and its exercise in communities is highly complex. The power to influence others may rest on the ability to give or withhold satisfactions from others in spheres not directly related to the immediate issue. A monopoly of oxygen on the moon, for example, would give its possessor absolute power over other inhabitants in every sphere of life, other factors being equal.

Ability to influence may be a function of the skill of the influencer and the methods he uses. Skill itself or the adequacy of the method become the resources possessed more or less abundantly by persons or groups. Energy and time are further examples of resources that, if marshaled effectively, represent potent wellsprings of power. Power may reside in the legitimacy of the argument itself or in the appropriate exercise of the authority inherent in an official position.

Thus power is neither absolute nor unlimited, even in totally authoritarian situations. Also, because there are multiple sources of power in the community, it tends to fluctuate, depending on the nature of the issue and the relevancy of the resources possessed by the individual or group. It is also important to note that not all power is manifest and actively brought to bear in community situations. Other power may exist as a potential force by dint of the intellectual, monetary, or other resources of the individual or group, even though it is not exercised at a particular time.

Obviously, power is in part a function of the perceptions of those involved. The charismatic leader, for instance, in reality may have little or no competence; it is enough that others perceive him as a resource. Power exists so long as it is invested in some person, thing, or group by those who are influenced by that power. The fact that most people have a simplistic, unitary perception of power in which those at the top of the heap are seen as potent and those at the bottom experience themselves as relatively powerless, contributes to a state of affairs in which power is largely expressed from the top downward. As witnessed in recent civil rights and antipoverty movements, those at the bottom do indeed have power, but it is mainly unexpressed and potential.

In community systems most roles and positions are complementary in that each member has power over another by virtue of the fact that the other's role is dependent on the readiness of each to reciprocate the relationship. In the words of the old cliché, "it takes two to tango." Power is reciprocal. The powerful role or position held by any individual or group is maintained by a complementary set of role relationships with those accepting the power.

Viguers (1956) has done an excellent job of portraying the plurality and complementarity of power. Although his description is limited to coexisting status hierarchies in general hospitals, it is applicable to a variety of community settings. According to Viguers, there are coexisting power systems each deriving its position from a different source or set of resources. The administrator of the hospital, by reason of his official authority, has the power to enforce regulations. The professional responsibilities and competence of a physician, however, enable him to ignore a rule if, in his opinion, obedience to it would be detrimental to his patient in a medical emergency. Similarly, the custodian who is friendly with the nurse in charge of a ward and has done many favors for her and her colleagues may be able to gain admission to the ward for a relative even though officially the decision has been made that the ward is filled to capacity. Whereas the hospital's medical director, by virtue of his position, responsibility and training, influences administrative decisions made by the administrator, the chief of one of the services, if he is the administrator's personal physician, may be in a position to exert special influence on the executive's thinking about the needs of that service.

When people are involved in community controversy, they often find it hard to recognize the existence of complementarity of power. They may, as a result, tend to ascribe too much power to the adversary or to themselves. I have noticed, for example, that in mental health we usually ascribe too little power to ourselves and too much to the opposition. Interestingly enough, the opposition on such occasions often projects on us a degree of potency verging on the magical. Such misperceptions are probably fostered by the fact that protagonists in mental health and other controversies usually come from widely different segments of their communities. They usually have not had the kinds of contacts that would enable them to deal with each other realistically.

It is obvious to the casual observer that power and social status tend to go together. The relationship is not inevitable, however. As Clark (1966, p. 12) has noted, the British monarchy today is but one example in human history "of high status that does not any longer come with the exercise of the right or the privilege of decision making powers."

It also happens that high-status groups enjoy a latent power to influence events which they rarely bring to bear but which is nonetheless potent when exercised. The positive sanction of one such person may ensure the successful establishment of a mental health program, if only because his power is so rarely brought to bear. Conversely, the determined opposition of a high-status figure can become a formidable obstacle because of peoples' tendency to defer to the high-prestige individual.

LINKAGE BETWEEN SYSTEMS

Mental health groups, together with political, religious, geographic, special-interest, and other aggregates, represent the multiple and frequently overlapping subsystems which make up the overall community. Relationships between these various groupings are as complementary as are those of individuals holding roles or positions within them. The specific nature of intersystem complementarity is to a large extent shaped by the ways in which subsystems are linked to one another and to relevant systems outside the geographic community.

Systemic linkage refers to the ways in which one system is related to another. Linkages also exist between parts of the same system. Within communities there are many points at which the various subsystems or subcommunities interact. We often speak of such subsystems as "the business community," "the religious community," "the health and welfare community," or "the political community." Though they maintain their own boundaries and their own inner distributions of power, social status, and the like, these and other subsystems (for example, ethnic and racial groups), overlap and are in continuous interplay with one another.

Interdependence. No doubt the various subsystems of the community are not linked as organically as are the organs of the body. Nonetheless they are obviously highly interdependent. The existence of one subcommunity often depends on the welfare of another. There are many ways, for example, in which the religious and business communities draw strength from one another, and both could not exist long without an adequately functioning educational or health system. The goals of all major systems must be sufficiently compatible so that coexistence is possible.

Many mental health centers are setting about the task of forging explicit inter-institutional programs based on the various obvious interdependencies between them and other subsystems of their communities. Schools, religious institutions, general hospitals, court systems and police departments, social agencies, public housing facilities, antipoverty programs, and health departments are prime targets. The task of translating implicit interdependency into explicit collaboration is often extremely difficult and requires continuous and thoughtful effort over long periods of time. The reasons for such difficulties are usually apparent only after the fact. One basic factor lies in the fact that whereas interdependence of the implicit kind rests fundamentally on a kind of finely balanced coexistence, inter-institutional programming can only be achieved through explicit collaboration, which must in some major ways upset the autonomous coexistence of both institutions.

The dynamics of one of the earliest attempts to forge a collaborative program between a mental health program (located in the St. Louis County Health Department) and three county school districts are analyzed by Glidewell and Stringer (1967) in an excellent case study. Problems arose in such areas as value differences, concepts of change, handling of confidentiality, control and authority, and even fundamental goals. Mental health workers were perceived as threatening "foreign bodies." Teachers were thrown into conflict when asked to respond to disturbed children's emotional needs with the attitudes and techniques of the mental hygiene clinic.

Twelve years after the school mental health program was initiated it was clear that successful linkage was finally being established. New roles had emerged, and new policies and postures established that enabled both the schools and the mental health program to retain their own necessary decision making powers in a framework of mutual acceptance of responsibility for the overall program.

More or less related to functional interdependence is a kind of *psychological interdependence* which exists between subsystems both within and between communities. Psychological interdependence is a cornerstone in the self-definition of any group, organization, subcommunity, or total community. Much the same as reference groups do for the individual, it relates each system to a number of others with which it is either compared or contrasted. The favorable or unfavorable comparative references to other communities made by residents of a particular locality usually reveal a great deal about their communal values and aspirations. Ask most people to tell you about their communities, and if you remain with the subject long enough they are apt to say something like, "Well, Boston is a wonderful cultural center. It has theater, symphony, and good restaurants just like New York, but the pace is less hectic," or, "People here are not snobbish, as they tend to be in Snootyville."

A familiar organizational example is the American Cancer Society (ACS). It is a national voluntary health organization, and therefore it is probably psychologically interdependent with other such organizations (Heart, TB, etc.) that compete with it for the voluntary health dollar and the loyalties of potential members. At the same time, it joins with the others in being equally interdependent with the various metropolitan United Fund organizations, because of some sharp disagreements that exist in philosophy and approach to fund raising, health education, and research support. Part of the identity maintenance of ACS would probably involve statements such as, "We are a national health organization, such as Heart and TB, but we do not go along with the United Fund approach to consolidated fund raising." It would be equally factual to state that ACS is one of a number of national corporations, but that, unlike business corporations, it is nonprofit. The first statement, however, is probably closer to the actual psychological interdependence of ACS than is the second. Therefore I would predict that a spokesman for the Cancer Society would place greater emotional investment in the first statement than in the second. The notion of psychological interdependence between communities and their subsystems is similar to Kelly's (1955) view of how personal constructs are developed and maintained. He pays attention both to the characteristics that are included or accepted as part of the individual's self-concept and those qualities which are excluded or rejected (the "not me's").

By exploring any community over time it is possible to develop a rough map of both its functional and psychological interdependencies with other communities and the interdependencies between its internal subcommunities. As suggested in the section on communication, the internal linkages between the professional practitioners, the political groups and social welfare leaders; or the religious groups and those charged with law enforcement (to cite two obvious examples), are both formalized and casual. Community councils composed of organizational representatives exemplify formal linkages; an occasional "spontaneous" luncheon of businessmen and welfare leaders illustrates informal linkage.

Few communities are islands unto themselves. As we have already seen, most of the major political, business, religious, and other subcommunities within any locality are parts of functional groupings that extend out into the state, region, and nation. Furthermore, geographic communities in sprawling metropolitan areas are increasingly confronted with the need for fostering linkage mechanisms for dealing with metropolitan problems.

An example of the necessity for geographic communities to come together for the examination of joint problems is the effort of other states whose minimum drinking age is 21 to persuade New York State to raise its minimum drinking age from 18 to 21. Connecticut and Massachusetts officials believe that such action would reduce the problem of automobile accidents suffered by adolescents who have been drinking, because it would discourage youngsters from driving across the border for alcoholic beverages forbidden them within their own states.

Communities also are finding that they need to develop means for coping with the impact of outside forces resulting from state and national linkages (Warren, 1956).

An example of the impact of outside forces is that of the Girl Scouts, a national organization with local units, which a few years ago elicited strong reactions within certain communities when it embarked on a revised organizational structure that seemed to place greater emphasis on regional than on local groupings. Such an action had repercussions not only for the local volunteer leaders within the Girl Scouts, but also for the other local community groups on whom Girl Scout units depend for financial and moral support.

The quality of linkages between local communities and state or national bodies is a growing and already crucial factor in the life of most localities. Taking the areas of social, health, and general welfare alone, it is apparent that almost all major developments affecting citizens at the local level in this country in recent years were initiated by and pushed from the state or national level. Most have necessitated increasingly close collaboration of local communities with state and federal governmental authorities. Recent programs of urban renewal and redevelopment are examples; so are most of the growing number of mental health efforts in local communities.

CHAPTER FIVE

Population and Environment

THE COMMUNITY AS AN ECOLOGIC SYSTEM

The systemic view of the community presented in Chapter Four has dealt with the community as if neither the characteristics of its population nor its environment affected its way of life. Of course this is not true. Although basic elements and processes are found in every community, environmental factors and population characteristics plus the values and traditions of the population have much to do with the problems it faces, the resources it possesses, and the problem solving approaches it uses. Clarity with respect to the ecologic interplay of population and environment is essential to the mental health team as it goes about the important task of determining mental health needs of a community and establishing program priorities and approaches best suited to that locality.

THE NATURE OF ECOLOGY

Ecology is concerned with the interrelations between one or more species and the habitats in which they are found. Human ecology focuses on the interplay between man and his physical as well as sociocultural environment. The word is derived from the Greek word for house, or, as we might say, home or homeland. In this sense the community is the homeland for a population, some members of which, for our purposes, may be regarded as emotionally disturbed by virtue of their physical or sociocultural place within the habitat.

An ecologic perspective in community mental health shares with medical ecology the view of health and disease presented in Chapter One, namely that rather than being states of the individual organism, they represent the process of adaptation wherein an organism and its significant environment are in a continuously shifting state of equilibrium and disequilibrium. The predicaments that confront large numbers of individuals and groups at various points in the life cycle occur because of the nature of the physical and social habitat. As we have seen, they are often experienced as sharp discontinuities forcing abandonment of previously learned role patterns and behaviors. They may result in intense emotional distress and more or less severe disruption of personality functioning. Thus the ecologic view emphasizes that for emotional crisis to occur there must be a convergence in time and space of certain environmental and organismic factors, so that the organism is in conflict with environmental challenges with which it attempts to cope in order to survive. By survival I mean, in this context, to include not only physical safety but also psychological security, the ability to cope, selfhood, and significance (i.e., the defining aspects of community discussed in Chapter One).

Much of a community's existence is taken up with the distribution and use of space. It can be said with only a little exaggeration that space is what a community is all about. Certainly the spatial distributions and configurations—the location of buildings, the defining of boundaries, the layouts of roads, the spotting of playgrounds, cemeteries, parks, and other open spaces—reflect the operation of the underlying dynamics of security maintenance, coping with problems, and according significance to individuals. Space is a precious commodity and, as we shall see later, man does not appear infinitely capable of crowding himself into a limited amount of territory. The ecology of space use reflects basic social processes and does much to shape them, thereby influencing the development of individual character.

Thus it is no wonder that some of the most bitter and prolonged conflicts arise in the community over matters of land use. Our feelings about territory and how we are oriented within *lebensraum* are at the core of our being. To be comfortably and suitably located in spatial terms may have profoundly positive effects on emotional well-being; certainly to be disoriented in space is associated with profound psychic distress and psychosis. Decisions about such matters as the location of superhighways through neighborhoods or the elimination of neighborhoods through urban renewal call into question both the basic security of the individual and his ability to defend his turf against others. His inability to influence such decisions reflects his lack of significance to the community and his marginal position within it.

The decision to destroy the old West End of Boston in order to eliminate slums and raise the tax base of the city generated fierce opposition among the urban villagers (Gans, 1962). However, despite some additional opposition among social agencies and a few politically influential people, the decision was made and the people dispersed. Fried (1963) emphasizes that in defending the West End against renewal, the people were not simply fighting for crowded, inadequate tenements; rather, they were desperately clinging to a home space that included the street, the neighborhood, a stable set of relationships, ethnic traditions, and key caretaking institutions such as hospitals, churches, and neighborhood centers.

A number of studies have demonstrated influences on mental health resulting from physical and social environments. I have chosen to mention some of the more important ones rather than to present a detailed account of the findings. The Faris and Dunham (1939) research was an early milestone in its careful documentation of relationships between the distribution of psychiatric problems and residence in certain characteristic zones of large cities. Following World War II, a number of ecologically oriented community mental health studies were inaugurated in the United States and Canada (Milbank Memorial Fund, 1953). They focused on such problems as the prevalence and incidence of both treated and untreated emotional disorders and resulting degree of impairment in different target populations (D. Leighton, 1956); the impact on mental health of the dynamic interplay between population segments within communities (Lindemann, 1953; Seeley et al., 1956); the emotional impact of urban renewal as a process of forced relocation and total destruction of an urban neighborhood (Fried, 1963; Gans, 1962); and the kinds of psychiatric help available to patients from different socioeconomic levels of the population (Hollingshead and Redlich, 1958).

More recently Kelly (1967) has been conducting a brilliant series of inquiries about ways in which differences in coping styles affect students' adaptations to high schools that present either relatively constant or fluid environments. In the constant environment students were unresponsive to newcomers. Hazing resulted when new boys' dress or manner were conspicuously different; deviant newcomer girls were ostracized and were the subject of gossip. A visible competence or skill in short supply enabled its possessor to be accepted provided he was willing to be dominated by the system. By contrast, in the fluid setting a welcoming committee oriented new students and even offered help to enable shy or reticent newcomers to make the grade. Kelly hypothesizes that maladaptive behavior in the fluid environment will be related more often to isolation and identity diffusion, whereas in the constant environment deviancy will be more related to acts against the normative structures.

It is apparent that such basic ecologic considerations as population density or dispersion must play a major part in determining how mental health resources are deployed. What works in a high density area of New York City (Peck et al., 1966) will not be the pattern of choice in a state such as New Mexico where population is widely scattered (Libo and Griffith, 1966) even though in both instances it is necessary to obtain assistance from persons untrained in traditional mental health disciplines.

More studies are required so that we can understand more precisely how the interplay between population and environment results in varying states of health or malaise. Nevertheless, there is no doubt that ecologic dynamics do indeed influence the rates of occurrence of emotional disorders, the ways in which aberrant behavior is defined by segments of the population, the means that become available for its treatment, and the effects on the community itself of the modes of intervention and programs established by mental health facilities.

By now it seems reasonable to conclude that many, if not most, psychological disorders can neither be understood nor controlled if we do not understand and have the means of influencing the interplay between the organism and the environment in which it exists. Although we lack much of the understanding and intervention skills we ultimately must have, we must proceed with extensive community-based and population-oriented programs not only because of social need but also to develop the ecologic sophistication that is essential. At the same time, however, research of a more basic kind is needed (i.e., not initially tied to mental health needs or concerns). We are badly handicapped by a lack of pertinent normative and detailed studies of the interplay between populations and their habitats. A noteworthy exception is the Barker and Wright (1954) description of the psychological living conditions and behavior of the children in a Midwestern community. These investigators are pointing the way to a growing field of psychological ecology and look forward to the mapping of situations just as today we map the physical areas of the world (Barker, 1965). A further step has been taken by a mental health team in Quincy, Massachusetts, which developed and tested a systematic schedule of questions designed to survey respondents' investment in and transactions with the major subsystems of the modern American community (Burnes and Roen, 1967).

Barker and Wright hope we will arrive at a time when psychological underprivilege and advantage will be as well mapped as economic levels. They are urging that we give far more attention than we now do to knowing more about the things men do in their daily lives and to plotting changes in psychological living conditions and behavior in as careful a way as we now keep records of changes in birth and death. Such a potential for the application of psychological ecology poses many questions for the mental health field, not to mention all of society. It raises specters of total planning and population control that are incompatible with democratic values and institutions as we know them today. Yet the intimations of these issues are already with us. Analytic studies of population characteristics are already important to social and economic planning on a vast national and international scale. Ecologic approaches are being applied by many groups for a wide range of purposes, some crass and some idealistic. Ecologic techniques are called on by businessmen seeking to determine future demands for their products, by church groups wishing to establish suitable locations for new parishes, by urban planners concerned with changing the physical characteristics of communities to meet new population demands in burgeoning metropolitan areas, and by world health authorities deciding on the optimal deployment of limited resources for the improvement of physical and mental health in underdeveloped nations. The futher development of psychological ecology should provide vastly more precise control wherever it is applied; the ethical concerns, which no doubt will become so urgent they can no longer be avoided, are already with us.

POPULATION CHARACTERISTICS

As has already been implied, an essential component of any ecologic analysis of a community is a descriptive account of its population characteristics and trends. Out of the enormous array of characteristics that are available for study, certain ones must be selected. Which ones should they be? Because mental health concerns are so closely tied to almost any aspect of community life, a persuasive case might be made for the inclusion of almost every conceivable population variable. Financial limitations make it impossible to be totally inclusive, and the problems of analyzing and retrieving relevant data speedily enough for the purposes of program development and modification would be enormous even if cost were no factor. Therefore, because of both practical limitations and theoretical considerations, it is desirable to focus any population-wide data collection. Some guidelines are provided by experts in the field. Spengler and Duncan (1956) present a threefold category system:

1. Certain characteristics have special relevance because they are known to be determinants of important processes affecting other population characteristics. Chief among such determining characteristics are age, sex, and marital status, which are usually readily available through the census or other means. They are included in most instances because

they affect such things as birth rates, migration patterns, and morality. In the mental health field, for example, it is well known that age and sex interact to influence the nature and distribution of emotional disorders and psychological disabilities. Among children, to cite one instance, the ratio of boys to girls brought to clinics, hospitals, school guidance facilities, and other centers for treatment of a wide range of emotional disorders is no less than two to one and for some disturbances is as great as four or five to one. The reaction declines in adolescence, so that in the adult age range the sex ratio is equalized or shifts to a preponderance of women for certain disorders.

2. Other characteristics are sociologic in nature and are important because they reflect and influence the socioeconomic structures of the community. Here are included such items as occupation and income, social and ethnic backgrounds, religion, and nationality. As has already been pointed out, the mental health field has many examples of interrelationship between socioeconomic characteristics and the kinds of emotional disturbance to be dealt with in a population, as well as the forms of professional help that are made available to those in need.

In addition, even the acceptance or rejection of the basic mental health program itself, as was documented for example, by the St. Louis County Health Department (Kantor et al., 1958) may be correlated with socioeconomic characteristics of different target populations in a catchment area.

3. The final group of characteristics includes those that reflect a kind of population quality, in that in each case it is usually considered desirable either to increase or reduce the level of that characteristic in the population. Among these characteristics are such things as literacy rate, level and kind of education, morbidity patterns, intellectual capacities, and the various other abilities (or disabilities) that affect individuals' performance of social and economic roles within their communities.

Having ascertained the determinant characteristics, the socioeconomic features, and the indicators of so-called population quality, mental health planners are in a better position to begin to determine their program priorities and to anticipate the problems and concerns they will be facing in a particular community. They also can establish some baselines to guide them in installing the kinds of record-keeping system that will help them to know what segments of the population are being served and whether attempts to reach untreated groups would be advantageous.

ECOLOGIC INSTABILITY

Few human communities in this era are in a position of ecologic stability. Populations are changing in size and composition; man's technological capabilities are altering the physical and, secondarily, the social environment. Old ecologic balances are breaking down because of increased mobility, capacity for destructiveness, computerized means for data processing and information retrieval, and enlarged communications capabilities. Competition for space within and between communities is increasing sharply, both because of population increases and because of man's greatly increased capacity for mobility and dispersal. Already we are experiencing consequences of concern to the mental health field.

Urban sprawl and the accompanying migration of relatively more affluent white families to the suburbs has resulted in extraordinary concentrations of working class and indigent Negro and other ethnic groups in the central cities. The widespread effects on the core city are by now widely recognized; they jeopardize the tax structure and enormously complicate the task of dealing with such problems as juvenile delinquency, family disorganization, and various forms of emotional disorders. Meanwhile, the post World War II concentration of comparatively well-educated, economically stable middle-class young families in the suburbs appears to have facilitated experimentation there with community mental health problems (Seeley et al., 1956) ; only a decade or more later were such programs attempted in the inner cities, where most of the serious psychological and social difficulties were located.

Mental health programs must gear themselves to accept and anticipate ecologic instability. To be even moderately precise, their predictions of future population trends must be based on a qualitative assessment of what human society may be like in the years ahead; it cannot rely on prediction based on trends that have occurred in the years immediately past.

The institutional patterns and established programs for mental health must be amenable to frequent change and open to elimination of old roles and services in favor of new ones. Emphasis must be placed increasingly on experimenting with new approaches, with far less reliance on approaches that have worked in the past or even those that remain applicable today but have little promise for tomorrow.

It is essential, I believe, that mental health teams search out the major problems of the future in the intimations of them which are part of the present. This is why antipoverty programs in some places are commanding the emotional and intellectual investments of a growing band of community-oriented people from the several mental health disciplines. It is also why the mental health field properly becomes engaged in support of Model Cities planning or the Peace Corps and its domestic counterpart, VISTA. My assessment of what the future may hold suggests that these and other concerns holding great potential relevance to mental health stem from two major ecologic processes.

1. The growing density and concentration of populations—fostered by industrialization, reduced infant mortality and improved general health care unaccompanied by equilibrating tendencies toward reduction in rates of birth—poses worldwide problems. They have been widely covered in newspaper and magazine articles and do not need to be analyzed here. My major purpose in bringing them up is to suggest that it would be a proper (and indeed urgently needed) allocation of mental health workers' skills if they were to become involved in such programs as planned parenthood, community leadership development, and the planning of urban centers to accommodate high-density populations in such a way as to reduce the sense of physical and psychological discomfort that usually attends overcrowding. (See the following material on crowding.)

2. The rapidly increasing dispersal of ethnic and national groups within and between countries is an ecologic process that brings with it a breakdown of previous barriers that isolated one group from another and reduced direct competition and clashes between them. Despite the efforts of believers in segregation, apartheid and nationalistic barriers, the old isolating mechanisms are rapidly being penetrated. This, too, is a challenge for the mental health field, which, in my opinion, should already be tooling up for a major mental health task that will become of critical importance in only a few years—that of assisting in the resolution of intergroup conflicts and of helping to discover new ways of facilitating trust between populations which, although widely different from one another, must cooperate and coexist if community is to be maintained.

CROWDING

Crowding as a form of ecologic instability in urban areas is a matter of increasing concern to the mental health field. Laboratory studies of animal ecology, as well as the observations by leaders in human ecology, indicate that sustained overcrowding of a species has profound and far-reaching negative effects. Calhoun (1962), for example, found that rats faced with sustained overcrowding suffered severe disruption of the usual patterns of social interaction. The death rate increased markedly, especially among females. Patterns of rearing the young were disorganized and sexual behavior became deviant in a kind of polymorphous way. Calhoun coined the term "behavioral sink" to denote the concentration of population that results when numbers increase in an enclave that, for whatever reasons, is not able to expand the space available to it. Hall (1966) suggests that the understanding of a complex problem such as crowding and its effects on human populations must be predicated on far more understanding than we now have of the ways in which we use and react to territory and space. He points to the fact that different societies go about space use in dissimilar ways. Western communities, for example, emphasize the linear relationship of streets, whether according to a radiating pattern from a central point (as in parts of Washington, D.C.) or in the familiar grid pattern. Japan, on the other hand, places the stress on intersection points rather than on the linear streets themselves. Houses in Japan are numbered according to their date of construction in comparison with other homes around a particular intersection area. Houses in our country, as we know, are numbered according to their position along streets. Furniture in some societies can be moved around within rooms in order to accommodate to shifting social groupings; in other societies furniture is treated as immovable. Walls in Western homes typically are immovable and spaces fixed; walls in Japan, on the other hand, can be opened and closed.

Hall also emphasizes the importance of taking into account social class as well as international differences in any consideration of crowding and its effects on mental health. It is possible, for example, that part of the problem of increased violence in some American cities is not the result of interracial tensions alone, but rather a function of the fact that people of markedly different cultures (i.e., lower class Negroes or Mexican Americans and middle class whites) are in contact with each other "in dangerously high concentrations."

Hall states, "Now even if it were possible to abolish all prejudice and discrimination and erase a disgraceful past, the lower-class Negro in American cities would still be confronted with a syndrome that is currently extremely stressful: the sink (popularly referred to as "the jungle"), the existence of great cultural differences between himself and the dominant white middle-class of America, and a completely foreign biotype" (p. 156).

By biotype he refers to the total world in which any species (in this case, man) lives, the world which man creates that, in turn, determines the kind of organism he will be.

Hall's formulation fails to take into account the social psychology of frustration and aggression, the gradient whereby previously oppressed people rapidly move from apathy to insistence once progress is being made toward amelioration, and the fact that, in addition to class differences, there are also real and tragic differences in the ways in which established institutions in our communities relate to black and white people. Nevertheless, his plea for a more sophisticated and multidimensional understanding of the pathology of overcrowding remains valid.

SUCCESSION VERSUS ACCULTURATION

The ecologist makes an important distinction between acculturation and succession. The former is the process whereby values and patterns of the community are passed on to newcomers (both the young child and the migrant from outside). The latter, more rare in human affairs today, refers to the series of steps over time whereby a previously uninhabited or so-called "bare area" is inhabited by a series of population groups until a stable distribution of population types is reached. There are many examples of succession in the history of American settlements. One is the by now familiar pattern of the development, over a few score years, of a fairly densely populated trading center from a wilderness settlement composed of only a few cabins. Another is the process, virtually continuous, whereby one ethnic or racial group succeeds another in sections of the inner city.

I am familiar with a small public housing project, consisting of about one hundred units, erected after World War II for returning veterans of a community. The first residents thus were almost all young, new families of veterans who viewed the project as a desirable first step during the time they were establishing themselves economically. Over the years, however, the more successful families have moved on. They have been replaced by a different population subgroup, namely older families in which the wage earner for some reason has been unable to earn enough to afford private housing, or broken families in which the mother is receiving welfare assistance. Population density has increased because the present inhabitants tend to have more children; the pride of belonging to a veterans' community has been replaced by a sense of defensiveness and shame at having to live there. Contacts with the rest of the community are reduced. Because there are fewer young veterans in the project, families there have fewer grandparents living elsewhere in the community. What contacts there are tend to be with agencies concerned with health, education, and welfare, and are most often focused on family problems and malfunctioning.

Thus we see that succession does not necessarily result in a highly integrated community. The resulting equilibrium may be based either on a set of healthy or pathologic interrelations within the area in question, and between it and other sections.

In most of today's metropolitan areas, however, both processes appear to be going on at least partially. Sometimes they are intertwined and hard to disentangle. Newcomers moving into an established community go through a period of acculturation during which they learn about and, for the most part, become identified with the beliefs and traditions of the area in which they have settled. Communities have ways of helping most newcomers with this process, though they often miss in the case of people whose previous traditions are felt to be quite alien and not open to assimilation. Mental health facilities in areas with high migration rates are in a position to aid newcomers both by helping them learn the skills of making the transition to the new community and by assisting the community to develop and strengthen its other facilities for absorbing newcomers.

Other newcomers, however, are moving into areas that have lost their previous inhabitants so rapidly that they are, in essence, part of a process of building up a new population in a previously "bare area." Massive urban renewal projects, in which large sections have been leveled and entire populations removed, are examples of such ecologic "bare areas." Rarely do the previous residents return in sufficiently large numbers to carry on old beliefs, values, and social customs. Moreover, if this is not enough, most such developments have been stripped of the stores, recreation centers, and a host of other amenities most of us take for granted. The newcomers there are not in a position to become acculturated because there is nothing to serve as a model for adjustment and there are few of the required basic supports. Years later, after new waves have entered certain housing projects, there remains a quality of disequilibrium and internal tension, which suggests that this habitat and its people have have not yet reached the point in the process of succession where a stable community can be said to exist.

I dwell on the distinction between acculturation and succession in order to emphasize the practical value to the community worker of an ecologic orientation. If the analysis presented above is correct, the objectives and the approaches to be used will differ, depending on whether one is dealing with newcomers to an established community or new inhabitants of an area that has not yet become a stable community. In the first instance the effort should be made to help the newcomers understand existing values and customs, to discover ways in which they can incorporate them with whatever modifications may be indicated, and to learn the skills needed to live according to the beliefs and customs of the new environment. In the second instance the population should be worked with on a more intensive basis in an effort to help develop primary group loyalties and to foster the creation of workable standards and values that will be supportive of the individuals and their attempts at forming stable interaction patterns.

VALUES, HISTORY, AND TRADITIONS

An essential part of the ecology of any human population, as distinct from other forms of life, is its reservoir of beliefs, attitudes, and values, which, as we know, are rooted in the history and traditions of the people. No attempt to comprehend a community is complete unless attention has been given to the beliefs and values it embodies. These may include beliefs and values held in common with other localities, others that help to give a special flavor and uniqueness to the community, and still others that, far from being shared by the entire population, are peculiar to specific subgroups within it.

The peculiarly American values and traditions common to most United States communities have been amply described elsewhere. Among them are other-directedness, the readiness to alter and subdue the forces of nature, and child-centeredness. Taken together with a commitment to action as against contemplation, these qualities have contributed greatly to the very development of the mental health movement itself. Mental health is optimistic; it brings people together with others in an undertaking which promises to tame human nature itself. Moreover, it is committed to the well-being of children. How could such a field, backed as it is with a scientific foundation and professional expertise, not receive enthusiastic support!

There are other values, of course, that lead some groups in certain communities to receive mental health programs with less than open arms. Among these values are an emphasis on the rights of the individual against the interference of the state and the inviolability of the family as the prime means of child rearing and socialization.

Although the major values and traditions of the society are found in all localities, there are differences from one community to another based on regional, ethnic, socioeconomic, and historic factors. These unique qualities will inevitably affect how each community deals with the issues and concerns coming within the purview of mental health. It is generally recognized, for example, that organized programs under the mental health banner have tended to be supported most readily by largely upper-middle-class communities composed of a high proportion of young families with children.

It is also important to recognize that most communities have developed patterns for dealing with problems and bringing about change. If the mental health worker becomes familiar with these patterns, he is in a far better position to accomplish his objectives than if he remains insensitive to local approaches. The differences may be as grossly apparent as the comparative readiness of some communities to go into debt to build public facilities as against others' insistence on a "pay-as-you-go" basis. Or they may be as subtle as differences in the use of such words as "problem" or "conflict," or in the readiness to equate "social worker" and "socialism."

In one community where I have worked the tradition had developed of holding neighborhood teas throughout the town in order to explain new social agency projects or gain support of a new community program. Women were usually more than willing to serve as hostesses and those invited usually attended, whether or not they were initially predisposed or hostile towards the project under discussion. This approach fitted in well with the community's traditions about hospitality and opening up its homes to newcomers and strangers. In another community, however, the traditions and values not only did not encourage but even actively opposed such an approach to community organization. Only close friends were invited into one's home. Attempts to organize a series of coffee klatsches to explain a new community development program never got off the ground. However, when meetings were called at public facilities many residents turned up. It is instructive to note that the coffee-klatsch idea had been proposed by a committee chairman who was a relative newcomer. It was not until such neighborhood meetings had failed that an old resident, questioned by me, revealed that meetings in individuals' homes were viewed with suspicion and resentment as taking advantage of friendship.

As long as the process of succession occurs gradually enough, there are powerful continuities of orientation within communities, despite the fact that individuals die or move away and are replaced by others. The new resident becomes identified with and accepted by the group only as he is able to assume those central belief systems for that group. Such beliefs represent what some have called a "community of values." Thus, when assessing a community, it is important to determine the extent to which traditional beliefs and customs have developed there, what the nature of the traditions are, the extent to which they have solidified or are amenable to change, and the degree to which they are shared by all or most of the residents.

It is also useful to know who the carriers of the community's traditions are. On whom does the community rely to pass on its beliefs and values to newcomers? What mechanisms are provided that the newcomer can use to learn the values and to demonstrate the extent of his commitment to them?

Often, the most strongly held beliefs or traditions stem from certain critical determining events of the past which engaged the former inhabitants at a deep emotional level and which have been passed down from one generation to the next. These beliefs originally were functional in terms of those past events. Sometimes, however, they become invested with significance in and of themselves, regardless of reality as defined by the outside observer. Whereas the preservation of shared beliefs, values, and preferred modes of problem solving may be reality based, congruent with the task facing the group, and meaningful as part of the maintenance of group cohesion, there are times when the maintenance of certain cherished values will actually impair problem solving ability and lead ultimately to the dissolution of groups.

A well-known example of the death of a community resulting from maintenance of cherished beliefs and customs beyond the point of their functional utility is to be found in the Shaker communities. These groups, pledged to celibacy, relied on in-migration, especially of orphans for whom they cared, as a means of maintaining their numbers. When social welfare agencies assumed the care of orphans and public health measures reduced the death rate among parents, this source of in-migration ceased, with the result that only a few survivors remain in what were once flourishing communities.

The above example well illustrates the tremendous potency possessed by community belief and action patterns under certain circumstances. By inference from clinical observation, it may well be that such traditional patterns are clung to most intensely when there is a sense of threat to the autonomy or equilibrium of the community. Experience also indicates that such intensely maintained patterns rarely yield to direct attack or rational persuasion, since they are of vital importance to the equilibrium of the individual or group. Some traditional community belief and action systems, as we have said, represent useful means of problem solving, past and present. Even though they are no longer relevant to the tasks at hand, they are part of the community's way of maintaining identity and cohesion.

A characteristic feature of today's scene may well be the reverse of the maintenance of traditions beyond their adaptive usefulness. It is difficult indeed to discover in today's communities the institutional and positional strongholds for the defense of tradition. Ministers are manning the barricades in radical assaults on the status quo. Even the school systems, long the transmitters of tradition, are being awakened to new responsibilities as major resources in the process of social change (Osterweil, 1966). Under the circumstances we may wish to consider ways in which mental health centers can be alerted to support the few remaining anchoring points whereby the more adaptive traditional values are maintained. In any case it is essential that the mental health team be alert to the values and traditions of the community, their roots and origins, and the extent to which they remain positively functional. For, as I have suggested earlier, the beliefs and customs of a community—though not as tangible as buildings, roads, or geographic features—are powerful, if not palpable, shapers of the lives of its residents.

3

Studying Community Processes

CHAPTER SIX

The Community as a Laboratory

It has been suggested that the community may prove to be "the ultimate laboratory" in which to study the institutionalized strategies man employs "to create a habitat which in turn shapes him."

BENNETT ET AL., 1966, p. 28.

Traditional sociologic research has yielded some useful views of community life. It has described the social and political fabric of communities varying in size, demography, economic base, and other characteristics. For the most part, however, the findings have consisted of relatively static cross-sectional descriptions that shed little light on the dynamics of community life. More recently, attention has shifted to community processes (i.e., to the interactional phenomena whereby inhabitants solve problems, adapt to change, and maintain characteristic patterns of integration).

Mental health research within community settings cannot slight either the cross-sectional or the process approach. Through the former it has been possible since World War II to develop considerable knowledge about attitudes toward mental health and illness and about the prevalence and incidence of mental disorders coming to the attention of hospitals, clinics, and private practitioners. At the same time, however, the greatest promise for the future lies in investigations of interactional processes as they occur in communities over time. This is so partly because we are now in a suitable position to carry out such studies. The very existence of so many new and ongoing mental health centers staffed by social scientists and clinicians enables teams of investigators for the first time in history to have access to significant processes in numerous communities and over long time periods.

Some of the most vital problems in mental health (e.g., the nature of help giving and help seeking patterns and the impact of emotional hazards on populations at risk) can be approached most productively through the study of interactions between individuals and the significant social environments over specific time spans. It is for these reasons that this section is concerned primarily with some of the operations that must be performed if process studies with community groups are to be carried out successfully without jeopardy to research efforts which may follow.

THE MENTAL HEALTH FACILITY AS A RESEARCH SETTING

What kind of community laboratory can be afforded by a mental health operation? For what kinds of investigations is it best suited? How can it be used to yield optimal results? Let us begin by acknowledging that few if any *a priori* limitations should be drawn around any laboratory. In fact, none can be drawn with any degree of accuracy or confidence. Scientific investigation is not always well planned. Discoveries in one sphere have frequently occurred during the course of investigations in a totally unrelated area; equipment and procedures intended to explore one problem may turn out to illuminate another one. All that can be claimed for the following discussion is that it presents one worker's view of the community laboratory as he worked within it. It is based on fifteen years of experience with exploratory research programs that have sought to clarify interrelations between the social environment and psychiatric disorders.

The term laboratory typically conjures up an enclosed area in which certain means for observing a specified range of phenomena are gathered. Usually there are arrangements for making systematic alterations in phenomena in order to observe their consequences for other phenomena. If this were the only or the best image, it might well be asked whether the community can with justification be termed a laboratory. The dictionary states, however, that the word originally referred to the workroom of the chemist. For myself, I prefer to regard the community as the workroom of the mental health researcher or any other social scientist seeking to study certain dynamic phenomena, just as the psychoanalyst's office has been viewed as the best and even the only laboratory wherein to observe and study certain personality dynamics. Adequacy of scientific observation is a function of the skill and training of the observer, but it is also a function of the setting in which observation takes place. In the experimental laboratory it is possible to make systematic observations under varying conditions over which the investigator has control. In clinical-medical research, too, modifications of experimental methods can be introduced, as when through double-blind procedures both patients and physicians are unaware that a specific treatment procedure is being used. In most community research, however, the relationship between those doing the observation and those being observed must often be less detached and controlled. Indeed, it is the unique relation between researcher and what is researched that to a large extent tends to define the nature of the community laboratory itself, the kinds of studies for which it is best suited, and the operations that are to be carried out if research is to be implemented.

Each of the social sciences has developed its own tradition of community research. Sociologists and anthropologists have carried out many community studies. Typically these are time-limited: the investigator relates to the subject population only long enough to collect his data, and his responsibility to the target community rarely continues beyond the period of the research. Sometimes there are repeated contacts, as when an anthropologist returns for successive visits to a primitive culture to observe the impact within the culture of diffusion of Western knowledge and values. From the experimental laboratory sociologists have derived certain values. In the first place, the intentions of the experimenter are hidden whenever possible from the subject in order to avoid bias. Again, the specific nature of the research is disguised through the use of indirect questions, projective materials, and other strategems. Unlike the experimentalist, the sociologist usually cannot expose his subjects to varying conditions; instead, he samples varying field conditions and relies on respondents who are encouraged to respond as fully as possible to the questions put to them. Typically the researcher frames his questions on the basis of some theoretical model he has derived from his reading and experience.

The anthropologist, too, operates within a theoretical framework, but he may relate somewhat differently to the persons he interviews. He is as often the follower as he is the leader in determining the precise nature of the questions he may ask or the observations he may undertake. He is used to relying on knowledgeable informants to teach him about their cultures. Thus his observations frequently represent the product of collaboration between researcher and informants, with much dependency on the authenticity of the relationship.

THE WELLESLEY EXPERIENCE

The following paragraphs summarize a ten-year research program conducted in Wellesley, Massachusetts by a mental health center.[9] From this summary it is hoped that the reader will gain a feeling for the nature of one kind of community mental health laboratory and the relationships with the community on which its studies were predicated.

This work was initiated by Dr. Erich Lindemann and a group of colleagues from the Harvard School of Public Health, the Harvard Department of Social Relations, the Harvard Medical School, the Department of Psychiatry of the Massachusetts General Hospital, the W. T. Grant Foundation, and the Community of Wellesley (Aberle, 1950; Lindemann, 1953; Naegele, 1955). A multidisciplinary team was drawn from psychiatry and allied professions, from sociology, social anthropology, and social psychology, as well as from epidemiology and other branches of public health. The task force sought to find ways to determine the basic community processes affecting emotional well-being, and to begin the discovery of effective techniques for preventing emotional disturbance and promoting psychological soundness.

Participant observation was undertaken at a number of points within the community. Explorations with professional and lay groups were begun in the areas of education, medicine, religion, law enforcement, social work, recreation, and community ecology and town planning. The clinical teams were made available to individuals and families with a wide variety of psychiatric problems seeking help to overcome life crises. At the same time, intensive studies of a small series of nonpatient families were undertaken in an effort to identify patterns of equilibrium and disequilibrium within small social networks (Lindemann et al., 1955; Van Amerongen, 1954).

As a result of preliminary explorations with schools and parent groups, the cooperation of some families with preschool-age children was obtained for a more intensive inquiry into the nature of parental roles and parent-child relationships in middle-class suburban families. Open-end, focused interviews with mothers and fathers were used (Aberle and Naegele, 1952).

[9] This summary consists of excerpts, with some revisions, from "The Human Relations Service as a Community Mental Health Laboratory," by Donald C. Klein, a report presented at the Scientific Session on Social and Community Psychiatry, on the occasion of the twenty-fifth anniversary of the Psychiatric Service, Massachusetts General Hospital, Boston, October 1, 1960.

Certain studies arose from a confluence of the goals of the mental health project and the interests of another group. School personnel, for example, wished to develop means for the earliest possible detection of children with incipient emotional problems. The schools, therefore, were readily enlisted in a collaborative longitudinal study of a group of children entering kindergarten in the 1950 or 1951 school year. The investigation, later extended to include all pupils in kindergarten and the primary grades, studied the children's adaptation to school and the possibility of foretelling adaptive and maladaptive patterns. This and other studies also sought to learn more about the nature and meaning of peer relationships in the preadolescent and adolescent periods as well as during latency.

Structured doll-play observation as well as psychological tests of the children and interviews with the parents about the children's social and emotional development and the current status of child and family were conducted with the 1950 group in the spring prior to kindergarten entry. Ratings by teachers, interviews with school personnel, observations of classroom behavior using a modification of the Bales interaction method, and sociometric ratings by the children were used at various points as their progress was charted during succeeding years (Gruber, 1954; Lindemann and Ross, 1955; McGinnis, 1954; Vaughan and Faber, 1952).

A practical outcome of this line of research has been the annual spring preschool checkup service to which parents can bring prekindergarteners for an appraisal of their social and emotional development. This program enables the service to detect cues of potential school adjustment difficulties and to forestall them where possible (Klein and Lindemann, 1964; Elizabeth Lindemann et al., 1967). Similarly, an extensive demonstration program of the South Carolina Department of Mental Health in Sumter County (population 75,000) has used school entry as a salient event around which to build a comprehensive preventive program (Newton and Brown, 1967). The project has developed and tested an assortment of interventions embracing "creative inaction," on the one extreme, to a total mobilization of available community economic, counseling, health, and other resources on the other extreme.

From the beginning various professional groups in Wellesley shared with the mental health staff their experience with a wide variety of emotional concerns. After cooperative relationships had been established, these groups became interested in participating in more systematic study of all predicaments coming to their attention during March 1952 (Devitt, 1953). A more intensive survey, which utilized refined methods of gathering and analyzing data, was carried out during April 1959.

These studies have helped to identify distributions of mental health concerns among the population of the town. They have revealed differential patterns of use of professional resources, both in regard to the nature of problems (whether social, economic, or emotional) and in regard to the characteristics of the populations served (Kaplan et al., 1956). Used in conjunction with area mapping of the community into homogeneous sections, the approaches to case reporting developed for the surveys appear to point the way toward identifying fluctuations in rates of occurrence of emotional crises and disordered relationships among population subsections. The hope is that as methods are further refined and as community confidence is gained, such surveys will become an intrinsic part of mental health operations in many communities.

The foregoing studies contribute to an understanding of distribution patterns and occurrence rates of difficulties within an entire population. They do not, however, pinpoint the natural history of disorders as they develop among population subsegments. For such a purpose a dynamic approach must be devised whereby patterns of adaptation of groups at risk can be studied over time during the period of hazard, extending from immediately before the introduction of the supposed stress to the time when the hazard is passed and equilibrium re-established. The prototype of this approach was to be found in Lindemann's study of bereavement (1944, 1950). Similar studies have been carried out in Wellesley and elsewhere since Lindemann's early effort. They have looked into the adaptive patterns involved in the absorption of newcomers to the community (Thoma and Lindemann, 1961), entry into nursing training (Rosenberg and Fuller, 1955), kindergarten entry (Klein and Ross, 1958), the birth of a premature child (Caplan et al., 1965), and hospitalization of a parent for mental illness (Rice and Krakow, 1966), among others.

THE NATURAL HISTORY OF EMOTIONAL HAZARDS

These and other studies suggest that there is a natural history of each category of hazardous circumstances. This means that each hazard:

1. Affects population segments at different points in the life cycle and poses challenges of a particular kind and intensity to individuals' customary adaptive patterns;

2. Is characterized for most people by a period of heightened tension during which their previous coping techniques are no longer entirely effective and must be modified;

3. Is embedded within specific matrices of sociocultural attitudes, expectations, and more or less institutionalized behavior patterns that determine how the experience impinges on those at risk and what resources are available for them to use as they cope with it;

4. Has its own sequence of adaptive problems that must be dealt with during its own circumscribed time span.

Such studies of emotional hazards contribute significantly to strategies of preventive intervention in the community, because they yield an appraisal of the hazard itself, the emotional reactions it engenders, the institutional arrangements and cultural expectations surrounding it, and the successful as well as unsuccessful coping attempts made by those affected. They make it possible to devise specific measures for assisting those in crisis, for helping them develop more effective coping patterns, and thus for reducing the number of casualties resulting from failure to cope with specific hazards. One instance is the study of nursing entry from which developed a method of group counseling during stressful periods, later employed with freshman nursing students at two hospitals (Rosenberg and Fuller, 1955).

MAPPING THE COMMUNITY

In order to discover patterning of predicaments and the use of caretaking professions one ingenious approach used a method for dividing a community into homogeneous neighborhood areas and subsections (Lewis, 1956). An outgrowth of collaboration between an anthropologist and a social geographer, the method relies on five kinds of information readily available from public records or field inspection:

1. The existence of natural or other physical barriers to social interaction (e.g., rivers, wide roads, high cliffs, woodland);
2. Assessed valuation of property;
3. Date of house construction;
4. Appearance of homes;
5. Distribution of major ethnic groups.

The resulting areas have been shown to have more dynamic implications for patterns of social interaction within and between sections than do the more usual groupings of populations by social class and socioeconomic status, or the clumping of populations within census tracts.

LINKING OF SERVICE TO RESEARCH

In the Wellesley experience research and service interests were linked together. The dichotomy between science and service no longer seemed meaningful in the kind of community mental health laboratory which emerged over time. The clinical, consultative, screening, educational, and other service activities contributed to the laboratory in several respects:

1. They represented the means whereby genuine and continuing interest in the welfare of the community was expressed, thus helping to maintain access to the population;

2. They identified phenomena and suggested hypotheses to be studied and tested more systematically through separate studies;

3. They served as the basis for selected action-research studies, wherein specific service activities became a means for testing one or more hypotheses;

4. They constituted "windows into the community" through which it was possible to carry out continuous participant-observer study of processes over time.

In its search for the most effective ways of working in the community laboratory, the Wellesley group used almost the entire gamut of available research techniques, including questionnaires, structured interviews, group interviews, observation of individual and group behavior under both structured and field conditions, analysis of public records, and participant observation. It carried out both cross-sectional inquiries and longitudinal studies of the development of a group of children over time. It employed epidemiologic approaches to the delineation of distributions of emotional states within population segments and to description of the impact of presumed emotional hazards on population groups. It studied total populations and used sampling methods where such approaches were impractical. It resorted to retrospective reconstruction of life histories of individuals and institutions, but also tried to make use of prospective methods when possible. The following chapters are devoted to two approaches that were central to the Wellesley work and that I believe to be basic to any attempt to delineate the complexities of an on-going community from a mental health perspective. These approaches are (a) dynamic epidemiology, and (b) participant observation.

CHAPTER SEVEN

Epidemiology and Community Mental Health

"Gone forever is the notion that the mentally ill person is an exception. It is now accepted that most people have some degree of mental illness at some time, and many of them have a degree of mental illness most of the time. This really should not surprise anyone, for do not most of us have some physical illness some of the time, and some of us much of the time?"

KARL MENNINGER, MARTIN MAYMAN, AND PAUL PREGER, 1967.

Epidemiology, the application of an ecologic approach to the study of disease, views a disease condition as growing out of the interaction between man and his environment (Gordon, 1958).

As the name denotes, epidemiology was initially the branch of medical science concerned with large-scale outbreaks of communicable disease. Today the epidemiologist is involved in the study of noninfectious ailments, such as heart disease, which exist "clearly in excess of normal expectation" (McMahon et al., 1960). In this category also belong the various forms of mental illness and emotional malaise.

The epidemiologic approach has at least three values for mental health research and programming: (a) it serves as a model for fundamental studies of the distribution of emotional disorders among total population, (b) it provides a set of guidelines for inquiries into the natural history of events, such as bereavement, believed to be emotionally hazardous to large numbers of people, and (c) it indicates ways of organizing studies of community needs and resources for the most effective prevention and control of mental disease.

The epidemiologist is concerned with the factors that contribute to the incidence and prevalence of the condition being studied among specific segments of the human race. His objective is to point the way toward methods of controlling the frequency of disease, particularly when an unusual outbreak is taking place or is threatened. He seeks to determine the manner in which a pathologic condition comes into existence within a population, the factors governing its frequency and distribution among subsegments, and its shifting pattern within the population over time. In the interplay between man and his environment (which is of prime interest to the epidemiologist) special attention is given to aspects of the physical and social environment that produce illness and maintain or restore health.

Epidemiologic methods include the descriptive counting of existing and new cases, as well as the rigorous discipline of analytic epidemiology, which seeks to pinpoint causal factors through carefully controlled studies of high-risk and low-risk groups. There is also the equally painstaking investigation of specific outbreaks of illness (e.g., food poisoning) in a single community.

PROBLEMS OF APPLYING EPIDEMIOLOGY TO MENTAL HEALTH CONCERNS

A critical aspect of the epidemiologic approach is its focus on entire populations. It is "concerned with the field observation of disease under natural conditions in whole populations" (Plunkett and Gordon, 1960). Having such a focus it is limited largely by the adequacy of access to populations, and more particularly by the availability of data about the condition itself. Epidemiologic studies of mental illness have become more and more frequent as general acceptance of the mental health field increases but, as we shall see, investigators are still faced with complex problems of access to essential data. There are also problems connected with wide variations in the definition of emotional disorders and the classification of behaviors associated with them. Studies are, however, being increasingly tied to denotable specific behaviors or events which can be measured or counted with reasonable reliability by different investigators.

In the beginning epidemiologic studies of mental disorders were confined largely to descriptive counting and determination of numbers of existing and new cases—usually of the major disorders requiring hospital care. In recent years investigating teams have turned their attention to methods that are beginning to yield a more accurate picture of the proportion of specific mental disorders in a population, including untreated as well as treated cases. This work has been seriously hampered, though not totally hamstrung, by the lack of acceptable criteria for the presence or absence of such disorders. The epidemiologist has said to the mental health researcher, "Tell me how to identify the cases and I'll count them." The mental health specialist in turn has been confronted by the fact that psychiatric nosology, only partially useful in hospital and clinic, to be sure, is of little or no value for determining the incidence and prevalence of cases among people not in clinics or hospitals. The question, "What constitutes a case?" is closely related to the equally sticky question, "When can a case be said to exist?"

Fortunately, some epidemiologists are somewhat tolerant of the inability of mental health specialists to answer the latter question because they have become familiar with the problem as they have investigated the many diseases with insidious onset, such as tuberculosis and the degenerative ailments. Despairing of pinpointing any definitive disease threshold for emotional disorders, many epidemiologically oriented mental health researchers have preferred to think of psychological soundness and malaise as ranging along a gradient of wellness. They emphasize that the full understanding of any condition involves the study of all levels of severity. Suicide can be used as a model for the gradient approach. At one extreme are the cases ending in death; at the other are the transitory mental depressions that are reactive and can be linked to the common emotional hazards of life. In between are the more sustained depressions that do not lead to physical attack on the self as well as the so-called "pseudosuicides" and the unsuccessful attempts by those who do not try again.

The concept of degrees of impairment has been an especially useful means for determining what to count and what not to count as a case. Though differing greatly from one another on the criteria for psychiatric diagnosis, mental health specialists with training in the method agree reasonably well as to whether or not a given individual shows a 10, 15, or a 20% deficit in ability to handle the responsibilities and challenges of life (Goldfarb et al., 1967[a], 1967[b]). Such consensus among experts enables the epidemiologic investigator to establish different rates of occurrence for several levels of deficit. This is an extremely promising line of inquiry in that it enables different research teams to carry out roughly comparable studies in communities of various types, sizes, and population characteristics.

A major methodologic problem in virtually any community study of mental health matters has to do with the determination of relevant population clusters on which investigation should be focused. One method of approach to this problem is to carry out comparative studies of two or more communities having known characteristics, as Leighton's group has done in contrasting integrated and disintegrated communities. Census tract information provided by the United States Census Bureau is often of great value for such studies in that it provides detailed demographic information about the inhabitants of each tract or area. Census tracts, however, are not so useful for studies of population clusters when the research is concerned with the identification of relatively homogeneous clusters. The method developed by social geographer Lewis (1956) (mentioned earlier) has greater promise as a means of identifying homogeneous areas within communities.

EPIDEMIOLOGIC APPROACHES IN MENTAL HEALTH

STUDY OF HAZARDS

The epidemiologic orientation is embodied in the growing number of studies of the commonly occurring life events which are apt to lead to emotional crises. I have already said that a number of studies of different emotional hazards have revealed that each has its own unique pattern and natural history. Duration ranges from a few weeks to six months or more, depending on the nature of the hazard. There are characteristic emotional and interpersonal patterns whereby individuals and groups attempt to deal with the situation. Also, each hazard has its own sequences of behavior and emotionality, some of which can be viewed as especially adaptive and therefore more likely to lead to reestablishment of equilibrium, whereas others presage more serious and lasting psychological disability. Epidemiologic studies of the many emotional hazards of living may someday form a solid basis of information on which more precise preventive operations can be designed for community-wide application.

INFORMATION ABOUT TREATED CASES

Data gathered for epidemiologic studies in mental health have been of many kinds. Coordinated statistical reporting systems within clinics and hospitals have fostered excellent comparative studies of the distribution of treated cases among different segments of the population in various parts of the country. Nonetheless, there are obvious limitations to the use of statistics based on clinical records, and much research, especially that designed to test hypotheses, must rely on its own methods for gathering information. With all their limitations, however, vital statistics gathered by mental health authorities within the states and nationally, when coupled with census information covering the whole population, provide the best available picture of the state of affairs with regard to those cases serious enough to require institutional care.

FIELD SURVEYS

After World War II the growing national awareness and acceptance of mental disease as a major health problem facilitated house-to-house studies using interviews, questionnaires, and check lists of behaviors and emotional reactions deemed relevant to psychological well-being. Such research has been conducted in a wide variety of communities, ranging from Nova Scotian villages (D. Leighton, 1956) to the neighborhoods of congested midtown Manhattan (L. Srole et al., 1962), and even to samples drawn from all the regions of an entire state (D. Phillips, 1966). The results are adding much to general understanding of the mental health picture in today's communities.[10]

Painstaking study of a representative sample of adult Americans living in a 200-block area of New York City yielded findings that tend to bear out less systematic observations of prevalence elsewhere in the United States. Nearly 60% of those studied were judged to be somewhat disabled by mental illness. Almost 25% were judged to show signs of marked or severe mental illness. Only 18.5% were found to be without symptoms of mental illness (Srole et al., 1962).

Respondents have proved willing to cooperate, perhaps because the teams doing such research have consisted of highly sophisticated community researchers drawn from the behavioral sciences as well as the mental health disciplines. Finally, some researchers have made use of key informants from the populations under study. These informants have been citizen leaders and members of professional groups in a good position to know about most of the cases of emotional disorder within their purview, including many not brought to the attention of psychiatric hospitals or clinics. One such study showed that *untreated* cases of serious mental disorder were more frequent in a middle-class suburb than in a lower-class urban neighborhood. *Treated* cases known to hospitals and clinics occurred more often in the urban than in the suburban setting (Kaplan et al., 1956). Within any single large city certain

---

[10] Some epidemiologists in mental health are critical of such studies on the grounds that, though prevalence data can be useful guides for mental health programs, these studies were biased toward overincluding physical diseases and symptoms presumed to be reactions to psychological stress, with the result that concern for minor disorders may siphon off too high a proportion of limited treatment resources needed for those with more severe mental illness within the catchment areas of mental health centers (Lapouse, 1967).

severe emotional disorders, most notably schizophrenia, are presented to psychiatric facilities at a rate three times as great for densely populated lower-class sections than for middle-class outlying areas (Dunham and Weinberg, 1960).

STUDIES OF SINGLE LOCALITIES

Some mental health programs, viewed from the epidemiologic stand-point, have represented intensive studies of the population-environment interplay within single localities. As mentioned earlier, the Leighton group carried out such a study for many years in Nova Scotia; also, Lindemann and his associates inquired into a single suburb and later into an urban population being displaced by a massive urban renewal program. These investigations reflect the special ecologic flavor of epidemiologic orientation—the focus on populations, the concern with the relationship between man and his environment, and the attempt to develop strategies of intervention based on the best available knowledge of the natural history of disease within the target population.

ANALYTIC STUDIES OF TREATMENT PATTERNS

When an individual becomes emotionally disturbed, what determines the facility to which he will turn and the kind of treatment he will receive? A study by Hollingshead and Redlich (1958) of a group of patients in New Haven suggests strongly that the social class of the patient plays a vital role. Not only do wealthier patients tend to be treated as outpatients by psychiatrists far more often than the less wealthy, but within the same institution, such as a public mental hospital, both the nature of the treatment and the profession of the treater vary with the class level of the patient.

Rejection of seriously disturbed patients by the community depends partly on the degree of isolation of treatment facilities from the everyday milieu. Observations of positive community involvement in patient treatment in England and Holland, among other places, have led to this conclusion. Moreover, the demonstrated inability of an intensive educational program in a Canadian community to alter attitudes toward the mentally ill reinforced the belief of those involved in the study that physical removal of the mental patient from his community both expresses and aggravates the fear of insanity prevalent in the general population (Cumming and Cumming, 1957).

When round-the-clock psychiatric emergency services are made available in large urban areas, they are used to a disproportionate extent by young men and women in their early twenties (Muller et al., 1967). This was true in such dissimilar communities as New York, Helsinki, and Boston. The fact that so many young adults spontaneously seek help from readily available general hospital programs points up the importance of such facilities to a comprehensive mental health effort designed to reduce the prevalence of lifelong psychiatric disabilities. Epidemiologic studies of referral, treatment, and disposition patterns should help us design and locate (both geographically and in point of available hours) mental health resources that can in fact be utilized by the populations they are intended to serve.

LONGITUDINAL ASPECTS OF EPIDEMIOLOGY

Time is an essential aspect of epidemiologic research. Any epidemiologic study has an element of longitudinal research within it. The very concept of incidence (i.e., the rate of occurrence of new cases over a specified period, such as a year), is itself rooted in the passage of time. This quality of epidemiology makes it especially promising for mental health work. Some idea of why this is so can be gained from a consideration of how best to go about reducing the number of patients in mental hospitals. This requires an understanding of the concept of prevalence, which in turn is directly associated with two other factors, incidence and duration. Incidence refers to the occurrence of new cases of a particular condition over a specified time period, such as a month or year. Incidence coupled with the period of time during which the condition in question is likely to persist (i.e., duration) yields the prevalence of cases existing at any particular moment in time. Most problems that have been of concern in the mental health field have tended to have low incidence but relatively high durations, sometimes extending over the remaining lifetimes of those afflicted. Such analysis has pointed inescapably to the conclusion that, initially at least, priority should be given to efforts at reducing the duration rather than incidence of the major mental disorders. Many imaginative programs have been developed that have reduced the period of time required for hospitalization, have returned mentally ill persons to gainful employment in greater numbers, and have provided, through aftercare services, means whereby those with continuing emotional problems can be maintained for longer periods of time outside hospital walls. The time perspective afforded by epidemiologic analysis thus has resulted in major reorientation of institutional care and related services.

Time also plays a part in the onset of physical illness. By comparison, however, it seems to be a more significant factor in the development of emotional disturbances. We know that, viewed retrospectively, the development of most such disturbances involves a continuity of events extending back into earliest infancy. Epidemiologic analysis, however, cannot be satisfied with such reconstructions. The retrospective approach has been shown time and again to distort the past in ways which make it virtually valueless for most research purposes. Retrospective studies, at best, are expedient substitutes. They provide approximate understandings of relationships between events over time. They must be resorted to where current observations of events during the period of time being studied cannot be carried out.

The most straightforward and satisfying approach, and unfortunately a difficult one for mental health research, is "cohort analysis." The approach involves the longitudinal study of a group of individuals who are born in a given interval of time, and are followed by means of successive observations over a specified period of years. A well known example of such an ambitious undertaking has involved a cohort of children born during a single year in Berkeley, California. Data collection bearing on the physical, intellectual, and emotional development of these subjects has continued to this day when the original children are, in turn, marrying and rearing their own offspring. Such truly longitudinal studies tap rich veins of information. However, they are very difficult to execute successfully. Rarely is it possible to maintain an intact investigatory team over the entire length of the study. Subjects move away, lose interest or in other ways become removed from the research. The masses of data that pile up over time threaten to be of a richness that defies digestion, though hopefully this sort of problem can now be obviated by the availability of sophisticated computer technology. The greatest difficulty by far is presented in the rapid and quite inexorable obsolescence of the theoretical underpinning and conceptual framework on which such studies are predicated. The Berkeley growth study, for example, began at a time when Watsonian behaviorism was predominant in the minds of most students of child development. Before many years the focus shifted to psychoanalytic ideas about human growth and development. Today's investigators may have the need to incorporate both the orientation of social system theorists and of the behavioral therapies stemming from operant conditioning theory. The point is that it is difficult and probably unwarranted to maintain a continuity of data collection based on a single conceptual framework over the entire length of a study concerned with the full span from infancy to adulthood. Thus one of the major benefits to be derived from the true longitudinal study is unattainable so long as the entire field continues to forge ahead both in sophistication of theory and subtlety of method.

Cohort studies of a more limited nature will give relatively precise comparative information about the incidence of various types of emotional or other disorders among different groups in a population. Hagnell (1966) reports a painstaking study (the first of its kind for mental illnesses) that was carried out in Sweden. A careful cross-sectional study of the mental health of a small-town population made in 1947 was repeated, with some modification, a decade later by different investigators. On the basis of his own diagnoses (he personally examined nine out of ten persons in the 1957 assessment), Hagnell estimates that one out of three persons will have manifested diagnosable emotional disorders by age 40, two out of five by age 60. Rates did not vary among people of differing socioeconomic status (in contrast to studies in the United States where inverse relationships are almost invariably found in prevalence studies).

There is yet another, perhaps even more serious limitation involved in the type of single cohort longitudinal study we have been considering so far. It concerns the assumption of comparability between any single cohort born during a target year and all other cohorts born in preceding or subsequent years. For a variety of reasons, groups of people born in different eras are probably not comparable with one another in all the respects most important for mental health research. Among other things, fashions in child rearing change rapidly and, so far, unpredictably from one era to the next. Shifts in population mobility, density, and other characteristics introduce alterations in family life from one generation to the next. Then, too, there are natural catastrophes, major depressions or periods of prosperity, great wars or sustained cold wars; all these must surely differentially influence the life situations of those cohorts born during different years. The comparative study of such cohorts should shed light on how changes in social, economic, and international conditions do affect the mental health of entire populations.

Epidemiologists have used considerable ingenuity in designing comparative cohort studies that, in whole or part, rely on information that can be uncovered in available records. Records of birth and death, clinical case files, police reports and court proceedings, cases of communicable disease (and other reportable conditions on file with public health authorities), records of school attendance and achievement, as well as a myriad of other data sources, have been pieced together by persistent investigators. It has been possible in this way to follow several cohorts over many years without having either to carry out direct and successive observations or to base findings on subjects' retrospective accounts. This form of prospective study, however, can be no more powerful than its weakest link, which is the adequacy and availability of relevant records.

At present, this link is weak indeed when it comes to most problems that interest mental health research teams. It is well known, for example, that most mental health concerns are taken initially to nonmental health sources of assistance, such as clergymen and family physicians. No mechanisms are now available for encouraging such caretakers to keep comparable records of the problems brought to their attention; moreover, present attitudes about mental illness and the need for confidentiality make it difficult, if not impossible, to develop systems in most localities whereby such cases would be reported to a central record system.

THE NEED FOR CONTINUOUS
CASE REPORTING

Without question, a most serious obstacle to the development of adequate community mental health programs is the absence of systems for continuous case reporting in a community. Even the most serious and prevalent mental health concerns (e.g., suicide and alcoholism) occur in our communities at unknown rates and exist in undetermined quantities (Felix, 1965). Under the circumstances, it is simply not possible to design, implement, and evaluate focused programs along these lines, despite the existence of such ingenious efforts as suicide prevention centers (Shneidman and Farberow, 1965) and programs of alcoholism control within large industrial concerns. A major shift in social attitudes will be needed before adequate case reporting will be feasible. Among those opposed to such a shift are many psychiatric workers who, understandably concerned, wonder whether case registry and similar reporting systems can adequately safeguard confidentiality of clinical data.

An outstanding example of what can be accomplished by painstaking systematic effort is to be found in Maryland, which has been in the forefront of epidemiologic research in mental health since the pioneer studies undertaken by Lemkau and his colleagues in the Eastern Health District (1941). In recent years the groundwork has been laid in Maryland for combining (a) studies of the demographic, social, and cultural characteristics of the population, (b) indicators of mental health status and role functioning, (c) inquiries into community perceptions and attitudes with respect to mental illness, and (d) longitudinal data about individuals cumulatively reported from a variety of agencies by means of a Psychiatric Case Register (Bahn, 1965).

There are only a few documented epidemiologic field investigations of "outbreaks" or epidemics of emotional malaise similar to field studies of food poisoning and other acute episodes of physical disorders in specific populations. In one such episode a team organized by the Louisiana State Department of Public Health conducted a systematic study of psychological, social, and physical factors associated with an outbreak of hysteria among students in a single school of a small town, during and after the occurrence (Knight et al., 1965). The report does not describe the interventions, if any, carried out by the team. Nonetheless, it is rich in its implications for consultations that could have been attempted with those implicated in the epidemic. The list could have included school authorities and parents, health officials, clergy, and law enforcement officers of the town, all of whom played significant roles in the outbreak.

Despite all the problems, however, there is no reason for pessimism over the long pull. Experience suggests that the very existence within a community of a population-centered mental health facility tends to focus attention on a wide range of epidemiologic dynamics relevant to mental health. It is the sophistication and orientation of the facility's staff that determine whether epidemiologic studies will be initiated. If the ongoing concerns of the center are about population-wide matters, then appropriate epidemiologic approaches become tools which are as necessary for its purposes as psychotherapy is for the psychiatric clinic.

CHAPTER EIGHT

Participant Observation and Other Methods

In contrast to the detached observer who remains outside the phenomena under study, the participant observer enters into the realm in which he is interested. He becomes involved in the setting in a role that permits him to interact with, experience directly, observe intimately and at first hand, and discuss with others involved, the events he is seeking to describe and understand (Bruyn, 1966). Participant observation lacks some of the precision of more controlled methods. It stands in contrast to the laboratory method, which is better suited for the study of things and impersonal events or those aspects of human behavior that are subject to measurement and quantification.

Despite its imprecision—or perhaps because of it—participant observation is a vigorous technique that is naturally suited to capturing the complex nature of ongoing and continuously shifting human phenomena. It is the method of choice in studies of complex social processes over time; it is especially useful in exploratory studies as differentiated from hypothesis testing and it enables in-depth understanding of phenomena that usually cannot be achieved by other methods.

THE PARTICIPANT OBSERVER ROLE

Participant observation can embrace a combination of approaches. It is, first of all, essential that the researcher take on the role of a member of the group being studied and that he participate in its functioning (Selltiz et al., 1959, p. 207). The role must be chosen carefully with an eye for providing access to relevant data, affording the maximum degree of mobility within the target system, and disturbing that system as little as

94

possible by the researcher's presence. If the role itself does not permit movement of the observer among all important aspects of the system, it must give access to key participants who do function within the otherwise inaccessible regions.

The participant observer not only observes close-up the interactions in which he is interested, but he also participates in them. Thus he relies both on his empathic ability, which gives him a feeling for the experience of others, and on his ability to experience and understand his own reactions. Participant observation does not entail only the systematic cataloguing of events, it also involves the effort to interpret the meaning of the events for the individuals concerned and to understand the social processes involved.

The participant observer has the additional tool of direct inquiry. Both through casual, curbstone conversations with fellow participants and through occasional more systematic use of questionnaires and other structured tools, he is able to search out the less obvious meaning of the events and to better understand how they are being experienced and interpreted by members of the target system itself.

In other field researches the investigator is able to maximize objectivity by interpositioning structures and devices between himself and what he studies. The participant observer, on the other hand, relies mainly on himself as the observing instrument. Therefore he must continuously calibrate himself and his own reactions in order to understand the events he is studying. Yet this calibration must be accomplished within a definition of role and relationships that are open to change at any time. On the one hand, he must have the flexibility and freedom to allow himself to function and respond freely to changing situations within the participant role he occupies; on the other hand, he must somehow remain as objective as possible, especially when his own behavior and its effect on the phenomena themselves is concerned.

Most workers in community mental health are schooled in participant observation, though few have called it that or considered it a research method. The psychotherapist is, after all, a highly skilled participant observer, and psychotherapy itself is a sensitive research procedure to the extent that the psychotherapist has skill in employing it for such ends. The psychotherapist must have skill in permitting the most free play of himself in this human interaction (at least insofar as his experiencing of himself and the other person is concerned), always within the precisely defined framework of a specific role relationship. The patient-therapist framework enables him to use his personal reactions as sensory devices in the interest of understanding and helping the other person. It focuses the principal attention of both parties on the phenomena most central to the patient and ensures that the therapist, in a partial sense at least, participates in the complex situation which he and his patient are seeking to study and understand. The same considerations apply to the participant observer in the community. The role must be carefully defined and clearly understood by all concerned; its prerogatives, responsibilities, and limitations must be clearly understood. Its locus within a social-psychological nexus must be developed wisely so as to facilitate observation of the most relevant phenomena.

The clinically trained mental health person has devoted considerable time and attention, in theory and practice, to the phenomena of countertransference and the importance of keeping in hand those personal reactions toward the patient that may destroy objectivity and impede efforts to help him. In addition to countertransference reactions, the participant observer in the community must also guard himself against possible distortions introduced by the tendencies, as familiarity grows, to identify with and become emotionally dependent on fellow participants. Those he is studying may become cherished friends; their travail becomes his; their joys are shared by him. Under such circumstances the sensitive observer is able to gain a richness of understanding that would be denied him by any other means. On the other hand, he may also begin to explain away or even take for granted certain phenomena that are at the heart of the system he is studying.

Care must also be taken in the selection of sites to be used for observation. It makes a difference where a worker stations himself as a participant. Different settings facilitate contact with certain people but not with others; some settings foster openness and informal interplay while others may illuminate more formal, ritualized aspects of the system. Since it is neither possible nor necessarily desirable to direct one's observations to all parts of the environment, a degree of selectivity is essential. It is only as sharp as the theoretical framework and intuition which guide it.

Kelly (1967) selected four sites in the high schools for time sample observations on an *a priori* basis according to whether the behavior would be affected by the setting or the individual, and whether it would be relatively open and spontaneous or restricted and covert. The sites were the principal's office (personal and public), lavatories (personal and private), hallways (environmental and private), and cafeterias (environmental and public).

In addition to role and site selection, it is also important to organize observations according to the dimensions under study and, when they exist, the hypothesized relationships among them. The participant observer, however, is often in the position initially of the naive naturalist searching for some inkling of possible patterns or relationships. The researcher, like the psychotherapist, must enter into the inquiry with a provisional set of ideas about the phenomena he is to observe and the directions in which inquiry may proceed. As in therapy, he must also take his cues from unanticipated events, modifying both the conceptual framework and research emphasis in midstream when indicated. As observations proceed, and he becomes more immersed in the culture he is studying, he should be in a position to specify more precisely what is to be observed, to develop more precise categories and recording methods for his observations, and to check the reliability of his data in some fashion.

The problems of reliability and bias can be approached in different ways. Usually a combination of approaches is required. The observer himself can make repeated observations of the same situations to satisfy himself that he has noted with sufficient accuracy events which were not simply chance occurrences. Two or more observers can be involved in the research in order to discover biases introduced by selectivity of the observer. The observer can be "debriefed" by interviewers from outside who are alert to possible distortions being introduced by the fallibility of the participant observer and the impact of the situation on him. When a team of participant observers is involved in a large and complex situation, it is possible for observations to be pooled and discussed in order to ferret out significant phenomena that otherwise might be overlooked.

In Wellesley the total staff, including special research teams, clinicians, and mental health consultants, met weekly for an entire morning to review in as much detail as possible events of the past week in which staff members had been involved or about which they had some information. Out of such piecing together of interactions within the community, frequently important leads and meaningful insights into patternings and processes of community life emerged. These meetings were rarely devoted to making decisions about program. Rather, they were designed to maximize possibilities for serendipitous discovery of unanticipated findings. Often, the presence of outside consultants or visitors not familiar with the project and the community facilitated the discovery. The apparently naive question of a wise person sometimes was the catalyst which enabled the staff as participant observers to view events with the intense freshness of the newcomer.

Control over bias of the participant observer is also introduced by the fact that he can check his impressions and interpretations with others involved in the situation. He is, in fact, able to ask those being observed how they view the events and even to ask them to react to his own interpretations.

THE CONSULTANT AS PARTICIPANT OBSERVER

Certain participant-observer roles lend themselves for use by the community mental health worker. He is, for example, readily accepted as a teacher by professional groups, parents, and others. Then he is in a position to learn much from those who come to learn about their community as it affects them. A child-study group meeting in a living room or nearby school may shed much light on the character and dynamics of the neighborhood. A course on child growth and development conducted for pediatricians may reveal much valuable information about how this group of specialists is understood and used by the community.

The role of mental health consultant is by now widely accepted and employed, primarily because of certain characteristics which make it of prime value for the clinician who becomes a mental health worker in the community (G. Caplan, 1959). First, it is manifestly a direct and straightforward means of tapping the clinical worker's knowledge in a wide range of situations; second, it permits easy transfer of skills from the use of self in a clinical relationship to its use in a helping relationship in the community. The role's value for community research lies in the fact that it gives the consultant potential contact with a wide variety of social and emotional predicaments, with virtually the entire spectrum of professional caretakers, and with individuals and groups drawn from many segments of the community.

It would be a mistake to limit mental health consultation as a research tool to the problems of case counting, inquiries into the distribution of mental health concerns, or other problems that are clinical or quasi-clinical in nature. The consultant as participant-observer can also be in a position to study more complex phenomena, such as characteristic role functions of specific caretaker groups, specific patterns of individual environment interplay that are conducive to emotional illness or the intricacies of community decision making in regard to questions and issues affecting mental health resources. To a large extent, of course, the kind of data to be gathered will depend on the nature of the relationship established with the consultees. The nature of the relationship is partly a function of how narrowly or broadly the consultant himself views his role. Take as an example the range of possibilities open to the consultant working with clergymen. Only a limited view of the role of the clergyman will be gained if the consultative focus is restricted to the consultee's work as pastoral care-giver. If, however, the consultant remains open to and curious about other aspects of the clergyman's multi-faceted role, he gains access to a wealth of data about community concerns, the church as a social organization, special problems of such groups as newcomers, single adults, adolescents and so on through a wide range of phenomena in the community.

When he is carrying out consultation within a formal organization such as the public school system, the consultant's access to phenomena also depends on the relative mobility that he is able to establish in the organization. Understanding of certain phenomena, such as patterns of authority, is not possible if he is denied access to all levels and parts of the system, or if he restricts himself to contacts only with certain groups such as guidance counselors or health personnel.

As suggested earlier, it is important that the consultant's responsibilities and the limitations of his role be clearly defined, not only to facilitate his success as consultant, but also to ensure the adequacy of his observations. By knowing the boundaries of his position, he can be more aware of, and correct, any tendencies he may have to become too much the participant or too much the observer because of his personal involvement in the phenomena being studied.

The consultant is a more effective participant-observer if he makes this aspect of his work known. Broadly speaking, there is a reciprocity possible in the consulting relationship. The consultant can from the beginning enlist the aid of consultees in the knowledge-building aspects of the role; as a result, both consultant and consultee can become collaborators in a scientific endeavor. Under these conditions it is possible and appropriate for the consultant to inquire into phenomena not immediately relevant to the problem brought by the consultee, or to establish contacts with parts of a consultee group or organization that, under ordinary circumstances, would not feel the need to seek his help. Having gained acceptance of the participant-observer approach, the consultant is in a good position to enlist the consultee's assistance in his inquiries.

NONPROFESSIONAL POSITIONS FOR PARTICIPANT OBSERVATION

Traditionally, the participant-observer role in social science research has not usually embodied help-giving or educational functions. Typically, the social researcher came as a sojourner and stranger, a visitor to the culture who has adopted temporarily some social role intrinsic to it, such as that of storekeeper. In most cases he has not come equipped with a participant role derived from his professional training. It does not seem unreasonable for the mental health worker today to follow the same pattern and to establish a participant-observer position independent of his core professional training. Indeed, some rewarding attempts have been made along these lines. In one case a sociologist, interested in the impact of urban renewal on a population, established temporary residence in the neighborhood. In another case a psychologist, studying the caretaking functions of policemen, traveled for several months in patrol cars on night duty in a large city.

The clinically trained observer seeking to become a participant observer of community processes usually finds his clinical training and orientation to be both an initial help and hindrance. He is aided by his understanding of unconscious motivations, intrapsychic conflict, and the many ways in which defense mechanisms function. Accustomed as he is, however, to assessing the individual personality, he often finds it difficult to perceive the individual in his social role within the complex networks of the community. With practice it becomes possible for him to integrate a diagnostic assessment of personality with an appraisal of the social factors impinging on the individual. His clinical sensitivities and skills then become adjuncts that enable him to be sensitive to the motivations and interpersonal dynamics with which he is confronted.

The participant observer is often dependent on the observations and assessments of others from the organization or community under study, for they have access to phenomena about which he may be unaware. They have direct and personal experience with events which he cannot experience even vicariously without their assistance. Yet if the organization member or community resident is too firmly embedded in the culture under scrutiny, he is too close to and too much part of the phenomena to be able to perceive and report them. Several authors have reported that it is important to secure respondents who are marginal to the culture in question. One of them (J. Dean, 1954) has identified three types of such marginal and therefore useful respondents. The first group, whom he calls "outsiders," are close enough to the phenomena in question to observe and report on them, while remaining outside the community or organization. Usually they are members of some other, related culture, social class, or organizational grouping. The second group, termed "nouveaus," are newcomers to the community or organization. Because they are in transition from one role or status to another, they are likely to be especially alert to the experience and therefore aware of the details of the situation in which they find themselves. Finally, there are the so-called "outs." Here Dean refers to the group of people in the organization or community who are contesting for power but do not have it. They are knowledgeable about what is going on and are likely to be willing to reveal discrediting information about those who are in power.

Generally speaking, I believe it is essential that all participant observation under the aegis of mental health centers be carried out openly and with full knowledge of those concerned in the community. There are instances in which researchers have apparently been able to ferret out otherwise unobtainable data by disguising their identity. The disadvantages and even long-run dangers of secrecy nevertheless outweigh any short-run gains. The disguised observer is unable to enlist members of the group he is studying openly and fully in his inquiry. He must guard against losing his cover by appearing overly curious, asking too many questions, or poking into situations where he apparently does not belong. More important as a reason is the essential distrust and absence of collaborative, shared inquiry that disguise introduces. If it becomes known that the mental health center (or any other group involved in community study) is engaging in secret inquiry, the existence of the overall program may well be jeopardized. The readiness of the community to engage fully in collaborative exploration of fundamental problems, in mental health or any other field, with behavioral scientists may be dissipated. Therefore an open, fully involving stance of participant observation appears to be the only practical way open to the mental health center.

OTHER METHODS OF COMMUNITY RESEARCH

The depth of observation and richness of texture afforded by participant observation are rarely, if ever, provided by other methods of community research. Other methods, however, are ordinarily more systematic, permit comparison of phenomena under differing conditions, are amenable to quantitative analysis, and can be more readily used to test particular hypotheses. For the most part, these methods are employed to examine in great detail a more restricted area of study; usually they concern themselves with cross-sectional views or with events over a very limited time span. Some idea of the range of information to be gained from these methods, as well as the variety and limitations of the methods themselves, was already reflected in the review of the Wellesley program.

Social research methods have been classified in a number of ways. For summary purposes in this discussion, they may be considered in terms of kind of data sought and the time perspective within which they are gathered. Simply stated, the social researcher relies on responses to his questions, observed behavior, or the public documents, and other records that are the by-products of the behaviors being studied. He depends on samples of behavior and observations of a portion of the population, or seeks to include all relevant behaviors and to study all members of the population. He may be content with careful observation of behavior in the real-life situation, or may get his subjects to behave in a more controlled setting. He may resort to face-to-face interaction with respondents, or may ask his subjects to respond to questionnaires or other instruments.

The focus of the researcher's interest may be on the interrelationship between variables at any moment in time, in which case he will seek a cross-sectional or snapshot view of the phenomena. On the other hand, he may wish to discover how phenomena change over time or how events occurring at one point in time may influence later ones, in which case his research becomes to some degree longitudinal. Continuous observations may be made over a limited time period, or data may be gathered, as in some epidemiologic studies, which show the interrelationships of relevant variables over entire lifetimes of a population.[11]

An unusual marriage of more conventional controlled research and naturalistic observation has been developed by Fairweather (1967) and demonstrated by him in the design of within-community treatment approaches for patients who might otherwise have been hospitalized. Having defined a social problem for which some innovative solution is required, the method of experimental social innovation proceeds to naturalistic field observation in order to identify the problem and its parameters in the actual setting. The action-research team then develops different solutions on the basis of the several plausible hypotheses or attractive action alternatives. The solutions, designed in terms of total subsystems (e.g., and entire classroom and curriculum designed to overcome the effects of early educational deprivation), are then tested experimentally to compare their effectiveness with other groups. The next step is to try out the innovations within their natural habitats (e.g., the public school system, which has demonstrated an interest in solving the problem of early educational deprivation) over the period of time needed to evaluate them properly.

Fairweather's model is an example of the fusion of action and research

---

11 One of the most useful presentations of pertinent research methods is to be found in Jahoda (1951). A more recent valuable text is Phillips (1966). Those interested in evaluation research (a complex topic which I have not attempted to cover) should find especially helpful a short monograph by Herzog (1959) and the detailed descriptions of the methods being used for evaluation of four mental health programs contained in a publication edited by Gruenberg (1966).

advocated by Kurt Lewin and later social scientists influenced by him. Many studies of small group, intergroup, and organizational dynamics have been enriched by the readiness of the research team to commit itself to interventions designed for bringing about solutions to real-life problems. It may sometimes be difficult, if not impossible, to introduce the degree of rigor and control required by Fairweather's approach. The multiple subsystems involved in most community problems and the complexities of community dynamics described in this volume will usually require the researcher to adjust his demands and rely more than in other settings on naturalistic observations. Fairweather's model, nevertheless, offers a useful standard and an important challenge.

CHAPTER NINE

Guiding Principles for Work in the Community Laboratory

Mental health research in community settings by now has suggested a few issues related to work in the community laboratory that may be important to the success of any research project undertaken in the community. Failure to confront these issues may jeopardize a project and even the community mental health facility from which it emanates. The following discussion of these concerns is based on the assumption that the research is being conducted by one or more investigators on the staff of a mental health facility located in the target community.

THE NEED FOR SANCTION

Each new research effort requires some form of sanction by relevant segments of the community, regardless of how well accepted the parent mental health operation may be. Among those relevant to the sanction-securing process are the board of directors of the mental health center, the professional and other groups in the community who may feel that the research is being carried out in their "backyard," and those persons responsible for the operation of other institutions or agencies in which the research is being conducted. Informed consent should be obtained from those who are part of the population being studied and from whom data are to be elicited, as well as from those responsible for them, such as supervisors, governing boards, top administrators, and parents. Once such sanction is secured the cooperation of subjects is usually assured; access to relevant background information is facilitated; and anxieties, which almost inevitably develop in the community in the early stages of research and which could become so overwhelming as to block the study, can be allayed by those whose opinions are respected.

Anxieties were aroused in a neighborhood when a researcher from the mental health center carried out on-the-spot observation of children's play behavior, despite the fact that parental cooperation had been secured. Neighbors called the school superintendent to find out what he knew about this suspicious behavior. Fortunately the superintendent was one of those whose sanction had been obtained; he was able to reassure the fearful citizens, and the research was able to proceed.

COMMUNITY COLLABORATION IN RESEARCH DESIGN

As it goes about securing sanction, the team may also be able to tap areas of felt need and identify questions that community groups would like to have answered. It may secure new information and leads that will suggest modifications in the focus or design of the study. This, of course, is especially true when the initial impetus for the research has come from the community itself. Even when the study is initiated by the mental health center, however, it can be advantageous to enlist the help of professional and lay groups in the consideration of such matters as the relevance of the research to the community, additional questions that may make the research of immediate value to it, anxieties that may be aroused and resistances that may develop, methods of data collection that will be acceptable, and additional sources of data that the research team might not have been in a position to identify.

In a discussion with a group of clergymen about a proposed study of the adjustment problem of newcomers to a community, it was possible to identify certain community organizations into which newcomers were readily accepted. The clergymen also suggested the Welcome Wagon representative as a source of information. Finally, the research team was put in touch with certain realtors known to have information about the turnover rates of homes in selected areas of the community.

SUBJECTS' PARTICIPATION IN RESEARCH

The foregoing suggestions propose a degree of openness and collaboration between researcher and subject not found in much psychological and sociological research today. Social science has taken seriously the findings of dynamic psychology concerning unconscious motivations and defensiveness. It has sought to develop indirect procedures whereby such motivations can be tapped and the defensiveness of respondents minimized. Subjects often are not being informed about the true nature of the research and usually little credence is given to their direct surface responses. Although biases may be minimized by such measures, the costs of deception often outweigh the gains. Relevant data concerning subjects' reactions and perceptions, which possibly would be forthcoming if the purpose of the research were understood, are not available. Moreover, the researcher-subject relationship may tend to reinforce already existing suspicions and anxieties about the nature of social research. Many people in the community believe (not without cause) that behavioral scientists view them as "things" to be studied; they suspect, too, that mental health workers have hidden powers of manipulating people. And there are those who are convinced that psychological damage may be inflicted if mental health personnel study them or their loved ones. The rigorous application of the laboratory approach to community research may exacerbate community fears and suspicions and has sometimes actually done so.

Although it cannot be demonstrated that the collaborative approach eliminates anxieties and suspicions, there is little doubt that it does often allay them. This is especially true when collaboration is obtained from the outset and community needs and interests are represented in the research design. The collaborative approach does not rule out the use of sophisticated procedures such as projective tests. It does require the researcher to convey the objectives of the research in an understandable way, yet in a fashion that will bias the responses and observations as little as possible. Having done so, the researcher is in a position to use whatever sophisticated approaches seem called for, including indirect methods of interviewing, observing, and even testing without sacrifice of either rigor or depth. If the principle of openness is not derived from the experimenter-subject relationship of the psychological laboratory, from where does it come? Probably it has more in common with the participant observer's relationship with the respondent in an anthropologic study or with the doctor-patient relationship in clinical medical research.

COMMUNICATION OF FINDINGS

After the researcher in the community laboratory has met the challenges already discussed, still other questions confront him. He now has multiple responsibilities to several groups of colleagues, the balancing of which can be troublesome. The problem of multiple and often conflicting responsibilities may evidence themselves in connection with the communication of research findings. In deciding on the nature, timing, and extent of communication of his observations, the researcher confronts obligations to many people who have a stake in the research. Among them, of course, are his immediate co-workers as well as his other colleagues in the parent organization. Then there are the subjects and all others who may have furnished relevant data. There are also the individuals and groups who have given the needed sanction which enabled the research to be conducted, or who have collaborated in planning and implementing the study. There is the community as a whole, which with its representatives' approval has been made available for study. Finally, there is the international community of scientists committed to the free exchange of the fruits of their labor. The issues involved here are complex; most of them are only now beginning to be explored, and it is not possible at this time to develop any sort of comprehensive guidelines. However, a beginning can be made by considering, in turn, communication between the researcher and each of the groups having some claim on his loyalty.

COMMUNICATION WITHIN THE
MENTAL HEALTH AGENCY

On the face of it, there should be no question about the exchange of community information between staff members of the mental health agency. They are colleagues, after all. What one has observed in his encounters with the community may help the others to make better sense of their observations.

We have seen that any community is a complex entity; its parts are so interrelated that a change in one is reflected to some degree in all the others. Although it is impossible for any one person to keep in touch with the interplay of community forces, it is both feasible and desirable for staff members to pool their observations periodically in order to tease out at least some of the most significant patternings and sequences of events. All members of the team, researcher and practitioner alike, devote their efforts to the same community, although they work with different segments of that community and with quite different specific purposes in mind. Their pooled impressions constitute at least a partial view of the total community gestalt, which stands as a backdrop to particular interventions and investigations.

Despite the advantages of such information exchange, open communication within mental health agency staffs is by no means automatic. Some of the difficulties arise simply because of limitations of time. Needs of patients, consultees, and others in the community usually assume more importance to staff members than information sharing sessions, which can become painfully tedious in the often fruitless search for possible interrelationships between events.

Far more weighty than problems of time and motivation, however, is the issue of confidentiality. This pertains both to work with patients and with nonpatients in the community. The ground rules for exchange of information between members of the clinic team are by now well worked out and generally accepted. Everyone knows that clinical data about patients can be shared with fellow clinicians and that there is every reason to assume that the patient's confidences will be respected and his personal predicaments treated with the objectivity and understanding that should be part and parcel of the clinician's orientation. With nonclinical colleagues, however, there is sometimes less certainty. Can researchers be entrusted with confidential information about patients? Should the research team and the community consultants be given open access to clinical records? Can the nonclinician be expected to understand and properly respect the patient's confidences?

The issue of confidentiality cuts both ways. In contacts with the various subsystems of the community, each member of the mental health agency, whether clinician, consultant, community organizer, or researcher, develops special relationships that must be predicated on mutual confidence and trust. In his contacts with consultees, fellow committee members, interviewees in a research, agency board members, and all other citizens, the staff member must assume the responsibility to exercise discretion in regard to what he communicates and with whom (e.g., Should confidences shared by citizens with the mental health consultants be shared with all other colleagues in the agency?).

Inevitable difficulties also arise over what information is relevant and what is trivial. Most of all, perhaps, who is to decide what to share and what to withhold?

There are no easy answers to such concerns. In general, however, I would urge that every effort be made to develop colleague relationships that will ensure that information of all kinds and from all sources can be communicated in the knowledge that it will be treated with confidentiality, understanding, and respect. This can be done only when the issues are faced openly and worked through to the point where each member of the team understands the responsibilities of the others to protect the rights and interests of their contacts, whether they are patients or not. Given our present inadequate knowledge of community processes, we need all the information we can get, and we need the investment of energy, time, and attention to the on-going analysis of the data flow as it comes into the mental health center. Later, perhaps, we will know better what to attend to and what to ignore. At this juncture it is far better to have an overflow of data than to run the risk of overlooking a pertinent clue or pattern of events.

COMMUNICATION WITH THE COMMUNITY

A different problem is presented by the desire of community groups to know what the researcher's findings are and what conclusions he has drawn from them. Is this desire legitimate? How should we respond to it? We know that such curiosity can arise out of anxious concern and defensiveness or voyeurism. There are other less neurotic motivations, however, that argue in favor of the feedback of research results, if only to those who have sanctioned or participated in the research. Subjects' participation in research, after all, represents an investment of time and energy. Moreover, participants sometimes place considerable value on the collaboration they have enjoyed. Their desire to hear about research results is a natural consequence of their investment and may be an expression of interest in maintaining the relationships they have formed with the mental health program. Furthermore, review of the data with individuals and groups in the community can yield new insights and interpretations, thus adding to the meaningfulness of the study. Also, citizens who have cooperated in research are often in an excellent position to consider and act on its implications for their community. There is a growing body of experience with community self-studies and feedback of research data which indicates that community research can be a potent instrument for bringing about change.

Finally, the most telling consideration of all may be that failure to communicate during and after research may result in reduced willingness of a community to participate in future studies. When the research team fails to communicate it is easy for a community to develop a distorted idea of what the research is all about. The resulting apprehensions can be quite powerful when it comes to mental health research. Many people, even today, remain convinced that "if you are not crazy before talking to a mental health worker, you certainly will be afterwards." Under the circumstances, openness of communication seems necessary in order to allay suspicion and distrust, and forestall reluctance to support future inquiry by the mental health team.

COMMUNICATION WITH THE SCIENTIFIC COMMUNITY

No one will deny that research is incomplete until a full report of the methods and results has been made available to fellow scientists. Unless such reports are complete and detailed, colleagues are entitled to have legitimate reservations about the value of the research and the conclusions to be drawn from it.

The requirements of scientific communication may come into conflict with the researcher's sense of responsibility to the community and the inhabitants who have cooperated with him. The inhabitants of most communities will have strong negative feelings about having the community's secrets appear in print, however professional and esoteric the medium of publication may be.

Social researchers themselves are in sharp disagreement on the question of whether information about communities can be treated as confidential or privileged. There is no generally agreed-on ethic concerning the publication of community studies. The usual practice is to attempt to safeguard the community by disguising its name and location, using pseudonyms in describing principal actors, and even disguising identifying characteristics such as occupation. These safeguards are probably effective with casual readers who may not be in a position to identify the communities referred to in such books as *Crestwood Heights, Middletown, Yankee City,* or the two small towns in Nova Scotia that Leighton called *Cove and Woodlot.* Such safeguards probably work well when social researchers study communities marginal to the mainstream of American life. Today, however, the mental health researcher finds himself among the organization men who live in the community described by Whyte or in the Canadian suburb depicted by Seeley in *Crestwood Heights.* Those knowing anything about the communities portrayed do not find it difficult to penetrate the disguises used.

Among the research worker's commitments to those from whom he gathers data is the promise, explicit or implicit, not to reveal information about the individual that may prove harmful or embarrassing to him. This pledge is easily honored when it is possible to bury the individual in statistical results. It is not so easily honored in some forms of study, however, such as those employing the descriptive case approach to critical events, roles, and relationships in a locality. Consider as an example a mythical but quite plausible study of the role of clergymen in dealing with alcoholism in a particular community. There are only a limited number of clergymen in any medium-sized community; often no two of them are of the same denomination. Suppose that one of them has himself been an alcoholic and entrusts the researcher with this information. The investigator is now faced with the problem of how to use and report this important datum. A possible "solution" is to disguise the identity of the clergyman in the report by altering his name, age, and other identifying characteristics. However, if the report becomes available in the locality, the clergyman may well wonder whether colleagues, parishioners, and townspeople have learned something about him that should not have been published. Undoubtedly, the rumor mill will grind out speculations that may affect other clergymen as well.

GROUND RULES USED IN THE WELLESLEY PROJECT

Recognizing the aforementioned problems, the Wellesley project at its inception established certain ground rules and procedures that have proved fairly successful. First of all, there was open discussion with community representatives concerning the need to publish research results. Problems of confidentiality were explored. The community people said frankly that they did not want to be "used" irresponsibly for the purpose of doctoral dissertations. They sought assurance that the findings would be published in a responsible manner under the guidance of the project director, whom they respected and trusted. Further, the community advisory board for the project made available a committee of its members to review manuscripts before publication and made suggestions concerning possibly unfavorable community reactions. In practice, no reports have been withheld because of community reaction; indeed, the citizens have been far more comfortable with publications than the staff had anticipated. After several years the anxieties of both citizens and staff were reduced to the point at which the review of articles and other reports became virtually *pro forma*.

Some research workers may object categorically to the involvement of community representatives in decisions regarding publication. Though understandable, such objections must be balanced by other considerations. It is granted that the basic obligation of the scientist is to his professional community and that when he withholds publication he does violence to that obligation. On the other hand, when, by publishing a controversial report, he arouses anxiety and resentment in a community, he does violence in a different way to his scientific obligations. He may be adversely affecting future opportunities for himself and his colleagues in the particular community, as well as in other communities, to carry out needed research. For the social sciences to prosper, there is need for a general climate of trust within the society. Otherwise the individual research worker will find it difficult indeed to gain the confidence of specific individuals who can provide needed data or withhold them. Anxieties aroused by one researcher in one community may make it difficult for another worker to carry out studies in another community (e.g., the accumulation of resentment over researches carried on with public school children in recent years has given impetus to efforts by persons hostile to social science to prevent social research of any kind in the schools). It may be concluded, therefore, that a responsible attitude toward scientific endeavor embraces the necessity to design, execute, and communicate research in a manner that will be harmful neither to the citizen nor to colleagues in community laboratories. In general, I believe we are in the strongest and soundest position possible when we approach these matters collaboratively with the communities concerned.

The training of mental health researchers is under re-examination in many educational centers, in view of the altered stance and enlarged perspective required of those undertaking community research. The adequate socialization of mental health researchers would ideally begin with experiences in the undergraduate years when young people are not so far removed from their own communities, rather than, as is the case today, during graduate and even postdoctoral education. Some of us have found, as Baler (1967, p. 251) succinctly puts it, that:

"Even senior psychologists enrolled in postdoctoral community mental health training programs often lack rudimentary practical knowledge of community organization, are totally inexperienced in operating in the real community in regard to sanction problems or collaboration with nonprofessionals, and find embryonic their mastery of relevant technical research skills, such as questionnaire construction, survey methodology, and the art of just plain naturalistic observation."

Fortunately there are within the mental health worker's repertoire some practitioner skills of relationship building, interviewing, and careful observation on which he can build his community research competence. Many of us are by now convinced from our own experiences that community research capacity, though perhaps attenuated after the customary graduate education, is by no means eliminated.

4

Change in the Community

"As our feet tread the earth of a new world our heads continue to dwell in a world that is gone."

G. S. COUNTS, 1961

CHAPTER TEN

Change as a Way of Life

There are grandparents in this country today who have experienced a shift from life patterns based on the traveling radius of the horse to the intercontinental span of the jet, from the communication potential of the telegraph to the instant culture and immediate participation of the television. As Hoaglund and Burhoe (1961, p. 411) put it in a recent discussion of evolution and man's progress:

"The mushrooming clouds of new notions and new patterns of behavior are altering the nature and circumstances of human life more within a few years than they were altered over centuries in the past."

Sweeping technological changes based on accelerating rates of discovery in almost all branches of knowledge are affecting community life locally, nationally, and internationally to an extent that cannot be grasped fully from this vantage point. The process is accelerating. Indeed, it is quite possible that, given the increasing rapidity with which major new influences arise, their full impact and implications will be understood only in retrospect.

From its inception, the United States has been committed to change as a way of life. Change was viewed as inevitable and desirable. Man's purpose, and for that matter the nation's destiny, was to prevail over obstacles, invent new solutions, and to remake landscapes when necessary to accomplish the desired ends of health, prosperity, and happiness. Though so-called "new-fangled" inventions inevitably evoked decryers, the inexorable march of progress went on. Even political institutions were designed with a change potential built in so that the constitution could be subject to modification by amendment as well as interpretation. The historic commitment to change was, however, linked to a set of principles which upheld the efficacy of spontaneous, unplanned, and uncontrolled adaptation to changing circumstances. A corollary to this principle of laissez-faire was that intervention during a period of adaptation could not solve the problem and probably would even worsen the ultimate adjustment.

Today the link between belief in change and the efficacy of unplanned adjustment is very weak:

"The progress of historic events has tended to undermine rational confidence in the principle of automatic adjustment as adequate to accomplish just, equitable, and desirable re-equilibration in persons, groups, and societies continually upset by accomplished or prospective technological changes" (Bennis, Benne, and Chin, 1961, p. 18).

It is true that there are groups that seek to uphold the principle of automatic adjustment, but their counsel seems increasingly to be viewed as an attempt to forestall further change or even to deny change when it occurs. The problem is that change today is both inevitable and rapid. Growing numbers of people believe that the American commitment to change as a way of life must be directed toward increased use of scientific methods for the purpose of coping with change itself. An indication is the growing body of literature pertaining to the planning of change and to the role of the change agent, the person who seeks to collaborate with those enmeshed in a problem in the attempt to find its solution.

MAJOR TRENDS AFFECTING LOCAL COMMUNITIES

Virtually everyone is aware of the great impact on localities of technological and other massive changes occurring in our society. Nonetheless it may be useful to review a few of the most significant trends before proceeding to a consideration of change as a process.

Five interrelated trends have been selected. Their combined effect on such matters as the ways in which decisions are made, the influence of local citizens on community affairs (indeed on virtually every aspect of community life) obviously is tremendous. Each change raises many problems; each presents potentialities for the development of healthier communities. The five are (a) the increasing relative concentration of political influence in urban as against rural areas, (b) the rapid development of sprawling metropolitan areas, sometimes called metroplexes, (c) the assumption by state and national governments of increasing responsibilities for health and welfare functions, including support of local projects, (d) the increased significance to a growing number of individuals of membership in various kinds of vertical associations, national and even international in scope, and (e) the facilitation of extensive efforts at comprehensive social and physical planning made possible by improved means for communication and processing of information.

FROM RURAL TO URBAN AREAS

The mass exodus from the land was associated with technological advances in agriculture and decreased demand for manpower on the farm. Urban industrial centers have expanded and multiplied as more and more people have entered their labor force. Although automation now represents a major new force that may bring the problem of human obsolescence to the city, the present picture is one of relative concentration of population and wealth in urban as against rural areas.

The struggle for power between urban and rural areas is an old one in the United States. It has played a major part in determining tariff, immigration, and other major national policies; it has been reflected in party affiliations and voting patterns of successive generations. The balance of political voting power generally has been with rural constituencies. Voting districts in many states remained unchanged despite population shifts, with the result that urban residents were under-represented in Congress, and rural residents over-represented. Nevertheless, the concentration of political influence in urban centers has been growing. The recent Supreme Court decision requiring states to alter voting districts in order to make representation more nearly equal seems to be a final step in the process of making urban power explicit.

FROM TOWN TO METROPLEX

As they grow, sprawling urban areas are invading the rural landscape. The children of the former farm families move out into suburbia, and businesses transfer to the industrial parks ringing the inner cities. Independent local communities, once fairly self-contained entities, find themselves caught up in a myriad of overlapping power, transportation, school, and other districts. Their inhabitants and leaders are struggling to maintain a sense of local identity and control in the face of new interdependencies with neighboring communities, and of problems that can no longer be met alone. Newly created localities, for similar reasons, face the problem of creating community loyalties and participation on the part of residents who look elsewhere for the satisfaction of many basic needs. Boundary lines between communities are less and less likely to be associated with open stretches of fields or woodlands. And, as many people had predicted, larger clusters of legally distinguishable localities are being blended, even across state lines, into sprawling intertwined metropolitan or regional concentrations of population. At present, these metroplexes are virtually formless aggregates of people and places, with no legal status and little sense of common identity or destiny, even among the leaders. There are those, however (e.g., the political scientists and planners), who look ahead to a time when the pattern of community government and human services will come to merge more closely with the major concentrations of population.

The growing interdependence of localities within metroplexes makes it necessary for those concerned with a problem to determine the extent to which it can be defined locally or to which it must be considered on a community-wide level. Moreover, the decision to treat one problem regionally must also take into account the inevitable impact on other problems and resources in the localities. Consider as an example the decision to consolidate two or three local school systems in order to arrive at increased academic excellence and diversity of educational opportunities. Such a change may have unforeseen effects on well-established collaborative patterns between law enforcement groups and educators concerning problems of delinquency prevention and apprehension of juvenile offenders. In such an instance, if the problem is defined simply as one of achieving a more balanced educational program, the chances are that related law enforcement concerns will emerge only after the change has been made. However, should the problem be enlarged in definition to encompass a more balanced set of educational and other services for young people and their families within a particular geographic area, law enforcement, mental health, family care, and a host of other variables are automatically included within the boundaries of the problem.

ASSUMPTION OF RESPONSIBILITIES BY BIG GOVERNMENT

The fictions of untrammeled free enterprise and of the completely autonomous individual who solves his own problems remain in some circles of our society. They remain despite the fact that in the past three decades state and national governments have been given responsibility for a variety of health and welfare functions, extending down into and affecting every local community. Millions of dollars are now being spent for control of disease, for rehabilitation, for treatment, for care of the elderly, for education, and for the poor. Although steps are taken to maintain a degree of local control of disbursement of funds and the like, it seems clear that groups of program specialists operating out of state and national offices are strongly influencing local actions and local policies. They do so through the allocations of funds, and, having granted money, through the settings of standards, consultations with local program personnel, and so forth.

Today, in many, if not most, metropolitan areas of the country there are a surprising number of federally financed projects of some magnitude which, often through the mediation of state governmental agencies, are carrying out planning and problem solving activities. These projects already are having major consequences, sometimes unforeseen and not always appreciated, for a host of local health, welfare, and recreational resources. State and local governments increasingly are bidding for a share of federal funds appropriated for attacks upon pressing social problems. Following World War II such money was committed to veterans' housing. By now there are contributions to area development, mental health, urban renewal, manpower retraining, delinquency prevention, support to higher education, aid to public schools, an all-out attack on poverty, model neighborhood development, and the list is not yet complete. The willingness to spend large sums of money through state and federal governments for planning and action extending down to the local community clearly reflects the implicit recognition that individual enterprise and local efforts alone are no longer adequate to meet the present and future needs of society. In fact, a major value shift may be taking place. Before, the primary emphasis was placed on local effort, to be reinforced only sparingly and when absolutely necessary by state and federal government. Now the primary emphasis is given to coordinated, centralized effort in which adequate funding commands the best scientific and other resources and directs them to the optimal solution of those problems for which an adequate amount of expertise is available. All other problems, for which there is no scientifically based approach, are left to the local community.

MEMBERSHIP IN VERTICAL ASSOCIATIONS

Ever larger proportions of people are becoming cosmopolitan in outlook. They are members of groups and organizations that cut across the bounds of geographic communities; their associations transcend the neighborhood or the local village; their values, attitudes, opinions, even behaviors, are shaped by inputs and loyalties unrelated to their immediate locales. There are increasing numbers of vertical associations available to and impinging on the individual. Lodges and service clubs, chambers of commerce, the parent-teacher association, nongovernmental national organizations devoted to political affairs, health matters, recreation, and the like, professional associations of physicians, beauticians, psychologists, training directors, and so on—a virtually endless list—all lay claim to the interest and support of the unwary citizen who ventures beyond preoccupation with his immediate locale.

In certain areas with significance for local communities (education and health are outstanding examples) policies and implementation of programs are already dependent on some form of accommodation between decision makers representing the local community and one or more critical vertical associations. For instance, the decision to establish a major new mental health program as part of the public health measures of the local community will usually involve the support of, or at least tacit acquiescence from, the county medical society, and certainly must be in line with policies established by the state health authority. The recent national debate over approaches to teacher accreditation, stimulated by the Conant report, also reflects the existence of multiple vertical associations impinging on each local community as it goes about providing education for its children. From the viewpoint of accreditation and sanction to teach, every classroom teacher is affected by a number of relevant associations; among them are the local school system, immediate colleagues, local, state, and national teachers' associations, the teachers' union (if it exists in the locality), the state educational authority that certifies teachers and establishes minimal requirements for localities to follow, and teacher training institutions (perhaps even parent-teacher associations should be included).

Often it is through their vertical associations that key groups within localities make it possible for outside influences to enter into the life of the community. A clergyman participates in a program on mental health sponsored by his national association, and several years later becomes the board chairman of a newly established mental hygiene clinic in his city. A health officer notes a growing emphasis in the *American Journal of Public Health* on preventive measures in mental health, and begins a series of steps which result in a mental health consultation program within his local health department. The examples could be multiplied without end, but the point is that vertical associations usually transcend local considerations when it comes to establishment of standards for scientifically based or professionally oriented programs, and for the initiation and alteration of such programs within local communities. Citizen bodies, such as boards and advisory groups, may make final decisions, but to a great extent they, too, are educated by their professional advisors to become oriented to outside values through vertical associations. Gouldner (1957) and others have commented on the prevalent split in organizations and communities between the so-called "locals" and "cosmopolitans." The former are epitomized by the inhabitants of old cultures wherein almost all attitudes and choices are shaped by inbuilt standards and values of the indigenous society. Residents of isolated small towns are examples, as are the "urban villagers" described by Gans (1962) in his study of the inhabitants of an urban neighborhood. Those living within vertical associations, on the other hand, are cosmopolitan to some extent in their relation to the local community. Bennis (1959) points out that the cosmopolitan derives part or all of his rewards from internalized standards. These, in turn, are drawn from his commitments to a profession, to a national movement, or some other internalized set of standards not subject to local pressure.

The citizen of the future may be one who is aware of the often divergent pulls of localism and cosmopolitanism. If so, he may be in a position to internalize the best features of both, without having to be torn between them. An objective of the mental health agency in a local community may well be to help the cosmopolitans among the professional groups respect local values, while encouraging the locals to develop increased trust in those whose values and behaviors are shaped by the outside.

COMPREHENSIVE SOCIAL AND PHYSICAL PLANNING

The era of the planner is at hand. Faced with massive, complicated problems, each of which must be considered in relation to others, it has become necessary for the society to direct some of its human resources into both specialized and comprehensive planning. The planner stands at the confluence of political science, economics, and architecture, with a growing input from the tributaries of social psychology and sociology. He deals with census data, production and consumption figures, tax bases, population trends, topography, mobility and other rates, construction methods and materials; he is increasingly forced by events, if not by his own predilection, to consider the irrationality of man and the needs and desires which, when translated into the vote, often make the difference between acceptance and rejection of this or that plan.

Planning, by its very nature, involves predetermination of an action or series of actions. It must be predicated on the establishment of one or more objectives, and therefore on determination of a system of priorities with respect to the use of human and material resources, time, and the like. Finally, it is oriented toward the future but must depend, for an adequate assessment of that future, upon complex data about conditions in the past and present.

Like the weather forecaster, the planner is no more efficient than the data available to him; for such data to become available in a meaningful way, they must be gathered, communicated, and processed. The burgeoning technology now available for data processing, storage, and retrieval enables the planner to make sense out of the most complex, multidimensional information. A major problem to which some planners are addressing themselves, with the help of behavioral scientists concerned with the planning of change, is that of taking into account the motivations, perceptions, and values of those people whose lives and communities are to be affected by the action plans. In a sense, this book is largely concerned with just this problem as it pertains to the professionals who are fast becoming planners and change agents in mental health.

CHAPTER ELEVEN

A Conceptual Approach to Bringing About Change

In Chapter Ten emphasis was placed on the growing awareness of change itself. The issue can no longer be—if it ever was—whether change should occur. Now the question is how such change can be met, shaped, and, when possible, anticipated.

LAISSEZ-FAIRE VERSUS PLANNED CHANGE

Reference has already been made to the laissez-faire doctrine of nonintervention in change. There is much that is attractive in this doctrine. Mental health workers committed to a belief in the inherent antithesis between individual well-being and social demands may well look askance at a growing reliance on social planning and a directed environment. Social scientists, aware of the tremendous complexities of culture, society, and the forces that shape them (not to mention the glaring inadequacy of present methods for studying and understanding social phenomena) may well question the wisdom of substituting misguided planned change for the natural social processes which nonintervention allows to operate.

Even with improved planning, technology, electronic calculators, and approaches to human engineering, how can any group take into account all that is involved in any projection into the future? No doubt the ecology and demography of a community can be expressed quantitatively; perhaps most of its functional qualities and how they are reflected in its major structures, even the patterns of communication and interchange of knowledge and beliefs, are manageable items for analysis.

But what of the attitudes, beliefs, and values shaped by the previous history and current situation of the community and its inhabitants? Can the actual and psychological interdependencies within and between communities be put into the picture? Given the complexities and the many factors which today must be placed under the rubric "imponderable," would it not be wise to allow the various changing factors to contend spontaneously and without interference in the market place until a new equilibrium emerges of its own?

The equilibrium theory breaks down when it is applied to conditions of rapid change. The analogy may be made to individuals and primary groups faced by an overwhelming stress or series of major crises. Under some circumstances the adaptive mechanisms prove insufficient to the task, so the individual or group regresses, in some cases even relinquishing any attempt to cope with the crisis. Marxian theory threw out the concept of an automatic return to an ideal equilibrium. According to B. Moore, Jr.,

"For a Marxist it is almost as difficult to conceive of a situation returning to a state of maximum harmony as it is for an equilibrium theorist to conceive of a self-generating cycle of ever fiercer struggle culminating in destruction" (1955, p. 112).

Ample evidence against the equilibrium theory is to be found in an era of cataclysmic world conflicts, the destruction of nations, profound depressions, and major revolutions involving millions of people. Marxism offers a conceptual approach to change predicated on massive and incisive intervention at the moment of grand crisis. Change is inevitable because conflict is inevitable within the framework of the class struggle. It is up to the architect of the change to shape the crisis and to assume the leadership at the moment when confusion prevails, and when masses of people are prepared to give allegiance to those prepared to act decisively. Such leadership emergence works, as studies of natural disasters reveal repeatedly. When there is crisis, old procedures no longer are sufficient to meet present requirements, and most individuals respond with dependence on any leadership which seems to know what it is about.

The alternative to the laissez-faire and radical-crisis approaches appears to be so-called "planned change." As defined by Bennis, Benne, and Chin (1961, p. 2), this is "a method which employs social technology to help solve the problems of society." As these authors conceive it, planned change seeks to apply systematic knowledge drawn from all available disciplines "for the purpose of creating intelligent action and change." The hallmarks of the approach are that change be (a) a conscious effort, (b) deliberate, and (c) collaborative.

Many of these principles are illustrated in a study by Blum and Downing (1964), who found that staff resistance to innovation in a community health center was greatest when administrative coercion was used and when informal patterns and existing status systems were disrupted. A three-person team for immediate intake and treatment of adults did not appear to have the total approval of the adult psychiatric clinic chief. Outside personnel were brought in to man the new service. Nearly half of the old staff resigned as a result. Complaints increased. Distrust of the administrator's motives was present in over half the staff, and fear, suspicion, and resentment were expressed by over eighty percent. A similar team was established within the child-guidance clinic, whose chief also had strong doubts about the move. In this case, however, the chief retained control of the activity, used inside staff, and integrated the program with the ordinary activities of the clinic. No staff members resigned as a result of the innovation. Complaints were infrequent, morale remained as before, resistance and suspicion were less extensive and disappeared more rapidly.

However, perhaps because of the departure of many dissident staff from the adult service, both innovations were implemented equally well. In fact, when each was absorbed within its parent unit, the adult clinic modified its procedures to become more like the experimental team's, whereas the organization of the child clinic remained as before.

RESISTANCE TO CHANGE

Those concerned with the planning of change must take into account certain endemic factors that tend to militate against either change itself or any effort to work toward it on a conscious, deliberate, and collaborative basis. The mental health field, in its clinical study of individuals, small groups, and even organizations such as mental hospitals, already has contributed much to an understanding of such opposing factors. To this body of experience can be added the findings of applied social scientists, such as Kurt Lewin and his students, who have carried on extensive studies of factors facilitating or inhibiting change in regard to a variety of behaviors. What is it that we can now postulate from such studies?

1. There is an almost universal tendency to seek to maintain the status quo on the part of those whose needs are being met by it.

2. Resistance to change increases in proportion to the degree to which it is perceived as a threat.

3. Resistance to change increases in response to direct pressure for change.

4. Resistance to change decreases when it is perceived as being favored by trusted others, such as high-prestige figures, those whose judgment is respected, and people of like mind.

5. Resistance to change decreases when those involved are able to

foresee how they may establish a new equilibrium as good as or better than the old.

6. Commitment to change increases when those involved have the opportunity to participate in the decision to make the change and its implementation.

7. Resistance to change based on fear of the new circumstance is decreased when those involved have the opportunity to experience the new under conditions of minimal threat.

8. Temporary alterations in most situations can be brought about by the use of direct pressures, but these changes are accompanied by heightened tension in the total situation, and therefore yield a highly unstable situation in which major changes may occur suddenly and often unpredictably.

PHASES IN CHANGE: LEWIN'S CONCEPTS

The process of change, as conceptualized by Lewin and most of those who have pursued the subject, involves three steps: (a) unfreezing, (b) moving toward the new level, and (c) refreezing at the new level.

UNFREEZING

Unfreezing refers to the condition whereby a previously stable state becomes amenable to change. It is analogous to the shift of a physical object from a static, inert state to a condition of movement. There is more energy required to produce the initial shift from rest to motion than to produce acceleration once movement has begun. For mental health purposes it may be useful to use the example of an individual seeking psychotherapy. When an individual comes for help there must be dissatisfaction on his part or among those around him with one or more aspects of his behavior or his situation. Dissatisfaction, however, usually is not enough, for there are various considerations that may persuade against recourse to psychotherapy. The cost may not be warranted by the severity of the problem or the individual may hold such thoughts as, "You have to be crazy to see a psychiatrist," or "Psychologists don't do anything; they just sit and listen to you."

At some point, however, there is a new input into the situation that enables the individual to unfreeze. These inputs are of two major kinds: (a) precipitants: events or circumstances that raise the anxiety level and make intolerable the status quo, and (b) facilitants: those inputs that remove critical obstacles to seeking psychotherapeutic help, without changing the nature of the problem in any essential way. An example of a facilitant would be the opportunity to speak with a trusted friend who has been helped in therapy.

As consultant to an organization of single parents I was responsible for arranging therapy groups for members. When members did not sign up for groups in sufficient numbers despite many expressions of interest, I was asked to write a brief article explaining the nature of group therapy and the kinds of problem for which the groups were intended. After the article appeared in the monthly newsletter of the organization, sign-ups increased, and it was possible to begin the program.

In most situations where people try to induce change, it is necessary to find ways to unfreeze the equilibrium. Complacency, hopelessness, self-righteousness, defensive self-justification, denial, blaming others or the nature of the situation—all these and more may confront those seeking to bring about change. It is important, therefore, for the change agent to be both clear and realistic about the nature of the desired change and the rapidity with which it is to be accomplished. In arriving at his objectives he must assess the resistances to be encountered and the steps needed to unfreeze the equilibrium and create the conditions whereby movement can begin.

The specific approach to unfreezing must depend on an assessment of the specific situation. A few general strategies are available. They include (a) provisional involvement in consideration of a situation, (b) direct confrontation, (c) acceptance of ambivalence through catharsis and support, and (d) creating a vacuum in the status quo.

Provisional Involvement. In this approach the individual is not required to accept the need for change in order to participate in the initial consideration of a problem. In fact, his participation may be enlisted just because he is convinced that no change is needed. The appeal may be to his willingness to keep an open mind or even to the desire to see that his point of view is well represented before any irrevocable actions are taken. This approach is most appropriate when those involved in the effort are able themselves to maintain a degree of openness about the supposed problem, and are willing to let the facts speak for themselves as consideration proceeds. The provisional approach is most effective when the definition of a problem depends largely on objective facts that can be viewed by all concerned with a minimum of distortion and screening through strongly held values and beliefs. It has the advantage of maintaining and even strengthening relationships and mutual trust between those who at the outset disagree about the need for change.

Direct Confrontation. Recognition of a need to change can be based simply on the clear communication of facts, whether the intent of such communication is to inform, alert, involve, or confront. Civil rights demonstrations, especially the initial sit-ins and bus boycotts, are an excellent example. They confronted the entire nation with the existence of a problem, and forced recognition of the unwillingness of Negroes to tolerate the present state of affairs. The situation became unfrozen and movement became possible when the need to change was recognized. Certain of the later activities of some civil rights groups, however, have been experienced by some whites as coercive attempts to impose situations on them, and, as a result, have been countered with massive resistance. (This is not to say that the strategy is incorrect; it may well be that purposes besides unfreezing are served in the eyes of the leaders and demonstrators, at this stage of the movement.)

The approach via direct confrontation may be most useful when large numbers of uncommitted people remain closed to change because they are unaware of the existence of the magnitude of a problem. Direct confrontation often does not occur *vis à vis* those in the best position to deal with a problem, namely those in positions of power and authority, because certain kinds of data are withheld from them out of fear, mistrust, or the unwarranted assumption that those in power must know what is happening and are choosing not to take action. Confrontation cannot occur if the assumption is made that the leader understands a problem and for reasons of his own refuses to take action. Without confrontation, the leader may be fated to remain in a state of ignorance and inability to act.

Acceptance of Ambivalence. This is the most nearly clinically based of the four strategies. It recognizes that individuals may be locked into a position of equilibrium because of the coexistence of opposed attitudes and feelings. While the wish to do something about a problem is present, it is countered by fear of loss of self-esteem or some other negative consequence if the problem is acknowledged and an attempt made to deal with it. Those faced with the conflict between their own prejudiced feelings toward a minority group and their equally strong convictions about democracy and fair play are examples of the kind of ambivalent "blockage" that is often involved. It is consistent with clinical observations to expect that sometimes those who are most vocally opposed to change are just the ones locked into an uneasy equilibrium because of ambivalence. The opportunity to ventilate feelings in an accepting, supportive atmosphere may represent the key to unlock the person and thus unfreeze the situation, whether in work with a patient or a community issue.

In the 1950's, when I was conducting a child-study course with a group of mothers from the Southwest, a rumor spread that a Negro housing tract was to be established adjacent to their homes. Subsequent sessions of the course were devoted to free discussion of the strong and universally negative reactions of the parents to the possibility. Various prejudicial attitudes were expressed. As the discussion leader remained accepting and interested, there gradually developed a shift in the orientation, and members began to express concern about the Negroes' reactions to the hostility and prejudice they might meet. After six such sessions, all but one of the group decided that, despite the continued existence of prejudices which they could not change, they would attempt to accept and live with Negro neighbors. Attention then shifted to how to forestall prejudice in their own children.

Creating a Vacuum. When the usual environment inputs are missing, customary coping patterns no longer suffice. Uncertainty and increased tension are created, with the result that individuals act to reduce discomfort. In the process, previously learned behavior patterns are brought to bear. Should these attempts fail, however, those involved usually address themselves to the unique problem confronting them. Action then gives way to appraisal, sources of information are identified, and new coping patterns become possible. The withdrawal of customary characteristics of a situation has been described by those engaged in human relations training through group participation techniques (i.e., the T-group) as "creating a vacuum" (L. Bradford et al., 1964).

The application of this approach to unfreezing has been tested extensively and found highly effective in human relations training groups. As used in T-group work, the approach elicits strong emotional reactions from participants; anxieties are aroused and there is apparent retrogression in behavior. All the evidence of crisis behavior is present. Considerable hostility may be directed toward the change agent as the training group works on such problems as trust and dependence on constituted authority.

Modifications of vacuum creation are used by all manner of change agents, from psychotherapists to community consultants who deliberately avoid responding with customary social clichés or in the customary patterns expected and frequently demanded by their patients or consultees. It seems clear that the vacuum approach is most feasible when the change agent is both perceived as a source of help and afforded the opportunity to remain with the situation during the period required for anxieties and hostilities to be worked through.

MOVING TOWARD THE NEW LEVEL

In a classic paper entitled "Group Decision and Social Change," Kurt Lewin (1947, p. 340) has pointed out:

"Any planned social change will have to consider a multitude of factors characteristic for the particular cases. The change may require a more or less unique combination of educational and organizational measures; it may depend upon quite different treatments or ideology, expectation and organization. Still, certain general formal principles always have to be considered."

As Lewin indicates, there are many specific processes involved in any instance and they are neither easy to observe nor readily analyzed. In the following, emphasis is placed on concepts and principles. More specific discussion of working toward change in community settings is contained in a later chapter on action models.

Establishing the Context for Movement. Lippitt, Watson, and Westley (1958) have broken down the "movement phase" of the change process into four steps, which they discuss from the point of view of a professional person who is attempting to offer help during the process of change. This individual, whom they call the change agent, works on (a) establishment of the relationship with the client system, (b) clarification of the problem, (c) examination of alternative solutions and goals, and (d) transformation of intentions into actual change efforts. Flowing from the initial definition of the problem, there are also decisions about whom to involve in a change effort and what kind of effort to mount.

The Context of Relationships. In any process of planned change, whether psychotherapy or community action, careful attention must be paid to the development of relationships with relevant individuals at all steps along the way. In most community situations considerable effort and time are expended in establishing trust and a climate for collaboration with a variety of groups. These may include lay and professional people within the community, representatives of regional and national voluntary and governmental bodies, relevant people from other localities, and with suitable helping resources.

In any condition of transition it is important to pay careful attention continuously to interpersonal relations and to the maintenance of trust and communication between the various groups involved. Collaborative relationships, once established, must be worked on if they are to be maintained. As change occurs, old communication channels may prove insufficient; new channels may need to be developed. Previous distributions of functions, responsibilities, and prerogatives may prove dysfunctional; they may need to be re-examined and altered to fit new circumstances. Ego needs of individuals and concerns of organizations about their ability to maintain member loyalty and achieve organizational goals must be considered.

In short, the adequacy of any effort to move toward change depends in the final analysis on human resources expressed not only in individual effort, but also in collaborative action within and between groups. During the period of transition, there are inevitable ambiguities. Resulting tensions and misunderstandings may impair relationships to the point at which available resources no longer can function. Both the professional change agent and those with whom he works will need to consider how best to work in the development, and how to maintain effective teamwork. Periods for consideration of the group's own processes and even the setting aside of blocks of time for more formal training in the sensitivities and skills involved in group work and community action have proved valuable to citizen groups working on complex problems.

The Context of Problem Solving. Three of the Lippitt, Watson, and Westley phases involve a basic problem solving model, entailing problem clarification, examination of alternatives, and implementation. More detailed consideration of problem solving in the context of social action is contained in the chapter on the development of community action. At this point only a few general points are immediately relevant. First, when people have entered into the phase of movement toward a new level, there is an almost universal tendency to express the problem in terms of some end product that is seen as the goal rather than the means. If people are concerned about teenage vandalism, the problem may become stated in terms of solutions, such as changing the legal age for drinking from 18 to 21. If people are concerned about reducing mental illness, the problem may be stated variously as, "We need mental hygiene clinics," or "There should be someplace where parents can go for help with their children."

Second, and closely related to the first tendency, is the desire to swing into action before assessment has been completed and preparations for action have been made. The inability to tolerate sustained ambiguity has often resulted in premature effort to attain concrete goals. As a consequence, the specific goals sometimes have not been reached. Or if they were attained, tension was reduced and pressure for action ceased, even though the original problem was neither fully understood nor solved.

Third, the problem solving context itself must remain fluid to some extent in order to allow the use of different resources and organizational structures that may be required at different steps along the way. Finally, just as in some instances groups may become prematurely committed to action, there is also a tendency for groups to avoid action. At such times clarification and examination of the problem become ends in themselves and the uncertainties of implementation are avoided.

Obviously, then, the development of a context within which successful movement can occur involves close attention both to the substance of the problem and to the human resources involved; to the structures needed to get the job done as well as to the creation of the kind of climate in which people may feel trust and support; in short, to the task and to the maintenance of the group working on it. Having helped create such a context, the mental health worker as a change agent is better able to help groups sustain the level of tension and dissatisfaction needed for adequate commitment to work on a problem, to avoid having to move prematurely to action, and when indicated, to make the shift from the diagnostic phase to the far more threatening arena of involvement in implementation within the wider community. Once again, the parallels to the psychotherapeutic process are readily seen.

The Dynamic Equilibrium. The field of planned change is also indebted to Lewin (1947) for a useful conceptual schema that can be used to assess possible strategies for change induction. Called force-field analysis, the framework conceives of any more or less stable situation as an equilibrium resulting from the action of opposing forces that are equal in strength to one another (e.g., a man who accepts the fact that he has an emotional problem but refuses to act on the suggestion that he seek psychotherapy). Assuming that he would not refuse psychotherapy under any and all circumstances, he falls somewhere along the continuum between total acceptance and total rejection of psychotherapy as a means of getting help for his problem. If all the forces acting on him were in the direction of securing psychotherapy, he would move toward that end of the continuum and would, in fact, seek help from a therapist. Conversely, if all the forces acting on him were opposed to securing therapy, or, stated in another way, in a direction toward total rejection of this form of help, he would entertain no notion of psychotherapy for himself. Thought of in terms of the goal to be sought in this instance, psychotherapy, the opposing forces have become designated as either "driving" or "restraining" in nature. The driving forces would be all those factors operating on the individual to move him in the direction of the goal of seeking psychotherapy; restraining forces would be all those operating to move him away from the goal (i.e., toward total rejection of psychotherapy). In this instance there could be any number of possible driving forces, among which might be:

1. Psychic discomfort;
2. Opinion of respected advisors;
3. Wife's insistence;
4. Crisis at work;
5. Relief to be gained.

Among the possible restraining forces might be:

1. Negative feelings towards a therapist;
2. Lack of experience with psychiatry;

3. Fear of insanity;
4. A conviction that only weaklings seek help;
5. Fear of ridicule by friends.

Because social forces can be assumed to be in a state of continuous variation, Lewin suggested that any equilibrium maintained by opposing forces would show continuous fluctuations around a level within a fairly restricted range. For this reason he gave the name "quasistationary equilibrium" to any situation in which the resultant of opposing forces is zero. For this kind of equilibrium to exist, it should be noted, any minor increase in one set of forces (whether driving or restraining) should be followed by a corresponding, compensatory increase in the opposing set of forces. Thus, in the example of the man considering psychotherapy, any increase in the driving force "psychic discomfort" would in a situation of equilibrium be met by a corresponding and countering increase in one of the restraining forces, such as "fear of exposure," or the impingement of a new opposing factor such as "the expense of treatment."

In developing a force-field analysis as part of planning change strategy, it is important to take into account forces that are latent in the situation (i.e., they will become operative only as the level of the equilibrium moves toward the goal). In the present example, negative reactions toward a particular psychotherapist could impinge at the equilibrium point only after the individual had secured some data about the therapist in question, either through personal contact or reports from others. Similarly, "relief to be gained" might become a far more potent force following an initial visit with the therapist. As Jenkins (1949) puts it, this kind of force is "one which acts as a driving force after some change has occurred," and is described by the statement, "If I can only get him started, I know he will find it helpful and will continue."

In the hypothetical example of the man considering therapy, then, the quasi-stationary equilibrium and its force field might be diagrammed as shown in Figure 2.

Obviously, many other forces might be at work in any such situation, including the relative accessability of treatment, favorable or unfavorable social stereotypes about psychotherapy held by the individual's key reference groups, the belief that one's problems are insoluble and fear that one's difficulties are more serious than they appear on the surface.

Using Force Field in Planning Action. It is possible to use force-field analysis to determine what modification of forces or factors in the community should be attempted in order to move toward a desired objective. The model simplifies the task considerably in that it permits a selection from among only three change strategies: (a) to increase driving forces by strengthening existing ones or adding new factors (b) to reduce or remove restraining forces and (c) to translate a restraining force into a driving force.

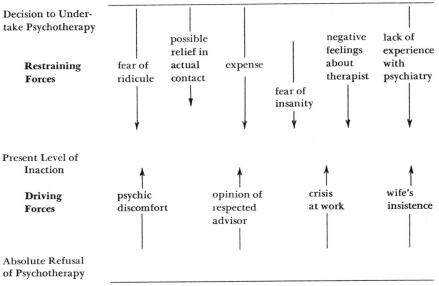

Figure 2. Quasi-Stationary equilibrium of individual undecided about entering into psychotherapy.

In many community situations, especially those involving conflict between opposing parties, the first strategy is most often used, as attempts are made to add to the strength of driving forces and to find new forces to throw into the fray against the opposition. When the thrust of such direct pressure is sufficient, the equilibrium level will shift. If all other conditions remain as before, however, the usual result is that compensatory increases in restraining forces ultimately offset the thrust and the equilibrium moves back to a point at or near the original level. The typical sequence of events in movements for municipal reform is an example. Immediate pressure for civic reform backed by the temporary mobilization of citizen effort often serves to "throw the rascals out" and "clean up city hall." Later, however, as zeal and enthusiasm dampen, the driving forces are reduced, while at the same time renewed efforts on the part of the "rascals" increase the restraining forces against civic reform with the result that the ousted group returns to power. Fluoridation offers an example of attempts to introduce community change wherein increase in driving forces (pressures from health groups) has typically resulted in corresponding increase in restraining forces (counterpressures from those concerned with minority rights and those opposing "forced medication"). No matter what the outcome in such cases, one result has been an increase in the total amount of force, and therefore tension, in the overall situation.

Lewin and others have noted that such intensification of the field is an inevitable concomitant of a change strategy based solely on the attempt to increase driving forces. When tensions rise in community situations as in clinical problems, the tendency is for the field to become potentially far less stable, with the result that sometimes sudden and often unpredictable change or acting out occurs. Under such circumstances, rational problem solving is replaced by irrational action based on emotional pressures and intense feelings of urgency. There are many examples in community life of such pressures and of attempts to deal with them. The provision of cooling-off periods in labor-management negotiations represents such an attempt. Here an institutionalized procedure introduces an anticipated reduction in the total force field by removing the necessity for immediate action. In dealing with family crises it is helpful on occasion to ask that decisions be postponed until after a series of consultations with the mental health worker.

A second approach involves modification of the forces that oppose the desired change. If driving forces remain unaltered, any reduction or removal of restraining forces will be accompanied by a shift of the level toward the desired goal. Simultaneously, there is a decrease in the overall force in the field, and therefore greater possibility for rational problem solving to occur if the tension level has been too high. In the example of the individual deciding about psychotherapy the opportunity to hear a talk on the nature of psychotherapy given by the director of the local mental health agency may provide a positive and safe experience with psychiatry that reduces a restraining force (i.e., the fear of psychiatry) and enables him to arrange an exploratory interview at the agency.

Finally, it may be possible to reverse the direction of one or more restraining forces. Such reversal, in effect, removes restraining forces and adds to driving forces at one and the same time. How can this be done? Using the example of the individual and psychotherapy, one of the restraining forces postulated in the analysis is fear of ridicule. Under certain circumstances, it may be possible to point out that the possibilities for ridicule are greater if the individual continues to ruin his life, while refusing the best available source of help. Or, in the instance of fear of insanity, another restraining force, it is possible that the individual may, if his symptoms worsen or a sufficient crisis occurs at work or in the family, decide that, without help, he will certainly "go crazy," in which case fear of insanity remains but now operates as a driving force, moving him toward, not away from, psychotherapy.

Some additional tactical considerations can be formulated on the basis of the force-field schema:

1. In most situations, the most effective approach appears to involve both adding to driving forces and removing restraining forces;

2. The most usual point at which adding to driving forces alone is effective is when there is need to unfreeze an equilibrium in order to make movement toward a new level possible;

3. While theoretically any of the forces in the field are subject to change, certain forces are more readily influenced than others. The most efficient tactic in most situations is to seek to reduce those restraining forces which can be influenced with the least effort;

4. Having determined which force or forces are to be influenced, it is important to analyze, in turn, the driving and restraining forces which will be involved in seeking to do so;

5. The process of force-field analysis, therefore, should be carried out repeatedly during the change effort. Jenkins (1949) points out that the process of force-field analysis is continuous. Having made intelligent judgments for taking action from a first analysis, the resulting action leads to change in the situation. Such a change to a new level of equilibrium itself calls for renewed analysis until the desired goal is reached.

REFREEZING AT THE NEW LEVEL

Lewin (1947) emphasized that it does not suffice to define the objective of a planned change in group performance as the reaching of a different level. Permanency of the new level, or permanency for a desired period, should be included in the objective.

The concept of transference cure in psychotherapy is predicated on the distinction made between transitory, short-lived change and a more permanent alteration in the emotional well-being of an individual. The attempt to introduce stability at the new level will rest on the quality of the remaining force field. As suggested earlier, if change has been brought about by direct pressure, restraining forces will persist. In such a case the driving forces that produced the change must be maintained in order to sustain the new condition. If, however, change has been accomplished by reduction of restraining forces, there is greater likelihood that it will be sustained without the maintenance of continued vigilance. The analogy can be made of the tense, defensive individual who maintains psychological equilibrium on the basis of continued vigilance against both id and environment, in contrast to the more relaxed person whose self-esteem and emotional security are predicated on a more manageable level of tension.

THE CHANGE AGENT IN COMMUNITY MENTAL HEALTH

Individuals, groups, organizations, communities, entire societies, indeed any dynamic system, are in a continuous state of change. Maturational forces, interactional events between systems, all of the manifold inputs from the changing technologies of the wider environment require that any organic system maintain itself in a state of continued readiness to adapt to altered circumstances. At the outset of this chapter, some of the more obvious changes confronting today's communities were reviewed. It was pointed out that there is often a dangerous lag between new inputs and the changes required to maintain effective equilibria. Because spontaneous adaptation often does not occur fast enough, there have emerged an increasing number of people trained in one way or another to help individuals, groups, organizations, or even entire communities as they work toward a goal of planned change in the function or structure of the system (Lippitt et al., 1958).

A partial list of such professional helpers or change agents would include all those directly concerned with mental health, plus others who can be crucial to the success of mental health efforts. Among them are adult educators, group workers, consultants within a number of professional areas, leadership trainers, applied social scientists, experts in conference planning, specialists in creativity, social planners, labor relations specialists, intergroup relations experts, community development workers, and extension agents. In addition to such professional change agents, there are individuals and groups of lay people who should be added to the list of change agents. Among them are the decision makers, those who influence policy, as well as less powerful people who, out of conviction, zeal, or personal need, work with groups and organizations to accomplish their ends in the community. Mental health workers so far have tended to cling to the role of the professional consultant-change agent who is brought into a client system from the outside in order to help temporarily with some mental health problem. There is reason to believe, however, that as mental health programs in institutions and communities continue to exist, there will be greater acceptance of the role of change agent functioning from within the client system.

The mental health agency, as it becomes more embedded within the community, will also be able to make increasingly effective use of professional and nonprofessional change agents from the community itself. It is even possible to focus attention on the development of built-in change agent resources within groups and institutions in the community. School systems, for example, are beginning to develop research and development teams. To help in the development of such intrasystem resources seems a highly appropriate function for any mental health agency since its overriding concern should be with the health-maintaining potentialities of the total environment as against taking on all or even most of such functions for itself. In most respects the elements of the collaboration between change agent and his clientele are to be found in the therapist-patient relationship. The change agent, like the therapist, (a) helps in the clarification of the problem, (b) enlists and marshals available resources (his own, the patients', and others') to help cope with the problem, (c) collaborates in the process of reducing the forces restraining change, and (d) remains with the client until an adequate new level appears to have been attained and stabilized. Unlike the typical psychotherapist, however, the mental health worker as change agent may not only identify a needed change, but also may become caught up in the process of bringing it about. Rather than waiting for problems to be brought to him, he may be a prime mover in the effort to unfreeze a situation, so that change is seen as being both necessary and possible by those with whom he may wish to collaborate in subsequent attacks on the problem.

CHANGE STRATEGY AND
THE NATURE OF THE ISSUE

If the mental health worker is to assume the role of active change agent, he must take into account the situation in which he finds himself, especially insofar as the attitudes and expectations of the several parties to the issue are concerned. Warren (1965) has made a valuable distinction among three points along a continuum concerned with the extent to which basic agreement appears possible. These are:

1. *Issue consensus,* where there is basic agreement as to the way an issue is to be resolved or where there is likelihood of reaching such agreement once the issue is fully considered;

2. *Issue difference,* where there is a good possibility that issue consensus can eventually be reached, but where disagreement exists either about whether the change agent's proposal constitutes an issue or about the substance of the proposal itself.

3. *Issue dissensus,* where important parties to the situation either refuse to recognize that an issue exists, or else they squarely oppose the change agent's proposal.

Warren suggests that in issue consensus, where the change agent is confident of agreement among the parties concerned, he can safely employ collaborative and consensus based strategies. In the second case of issue difference, where he does not have agreement but expects to get it, he will ordinarily be expected to resort to campaign strategies based, in part at least, on attempts at persuasion. In the third instance, issue dissensus, where he does not have agreement and does not expect to get it, he will ordinarily fall back on contest strategies that attempt to further his own side despite opposition, which he deems to be inevitable. Warren's analysis has the value of enlarging the concept of the change agent, originally developed substantially within the consensus framework, to embrace other prevalent change situations. The change agent now becomes not only the enabler or catalyst, helping a group reach its own consensus on the issue at hand; he also takes on the role of persuader, using mass media, face-to-face contact, organizational techniques, and so forth, in order to campaign for his proposals. Finally, he may line up as a contestant on one side of a community controversy or conflict, seeking to win against, rather than persuade or "win over," the opposition.

CHAPTER TWELVE

Can Community Change Be Collaborative?

ARGUMENTS AGAINST CITIZEN PARTICIPATION

It is no doubt apparent that a strong preference for collaborative approaches to change at all levels of community life runs through this book. Some may disagree with this bias, finding it at best the manifestation of well-intentioned, though totally impractical, idealism. Certainly there are many arguments to support the thesis that the local citizen cannot and should not, except indirectly through his elected representatives, be involved in the decisions that will determine the shape and character of the environment in which he finds himself. In such a field as mental health, it can be held, the citizen cannot become expert enough to make the proper decisions. He cannot take the time to inform himself even if he were able to comprehend the essential facts; moreover, he views problems from a too-personal and biased perspective. He simply does not have the technical competence and skill to make determinations in such spheres as mental health, urban renewal, and fluoridation of water supplies; therefore, all such matters should be left to experts.

Other considerations also argue against collaborative approaches to community change. Involvement of local groups takes precious time; change can be blocked entirely if agreements cannot be reached among local factions; besides, those with the power to make change and shape events are not apt to involve others in the change process unless those in power believe it is in their interest to do so.

Authoritative change, planned and implemented by experts, has many attractions. It is more likely to be quick, rational, based on scientifically developed information, and less distorted by local biases or individual prejudices. In short, it offers the security of authority and expertise.

THE CASE FOR COLLABORATION WITH CITIZENS

Unfortunately, however, "top-down" change also contributes to the weakening of community, for it tends to contribute to insecurity by bringing the control of events outside the citizen's sphere of influence. In the short run authoritative change may bring about community improvement and solve community problems. In the long run, however, a reliance on the authority from the top can have serious consequences for community life. The basis for this belief is the definition of community advanced at the outset: that it is an interactive domain whose inhabitants are concerned with security and safety, significance, and finding the solutions to the many problems of living. An individual's life today can be affected overnight in massive ways by decisions to remake the physical characteristics and institutions of his environment. When these are brought about without involvement either of himself or of those whom he trusts, the community (in the eyes of the citizen) becomes less secure and safe, less concerned with his significance, and more fraught with uncertainties that are added to all the other problems of life. There are many instances of community conflict and disruption of needed programs to show that the alienation of the individual weakens the community. In my opinion it also renders the individual more vulnerable to the kinds of social and emotional malaise with which the mental health field is most concerned.

A persuasive and research-grounded thesis that collaborative processes are inextricably interrelated with the promotion of mental health has been presented by Lippitt (1965). He also presents evidence that specific social interventions, based on knowledge of organizational and group dynamics, can be used to forestall authoritarian patterns and damaging conflicts.

For the preceding reasons I believe that the mental health worker should concern himself with *how* decisions are made in his community and with the consequences for the community of the ways in which changes are engineered; he should be prepared to intervene in an effort to influence change processes when, in his opinion, the community is being affected adversely (e.g., when those most directly affected are not being involved in the decisional process). He will be able to do so more intelligently and effectively if he has some comprehension of the complex hierarchical network of organizations and political jurisdictions in which any community exists today.

THE EFFECTS OF OUTSIDE FORCES

Local communities stand at the base of a number of major pyramids, consisting of groups and organizations that possess unique goals, values, responsibilities, and ways of proceeding to their ends. Big government, big business, big religion, big voluntary associations, and other major national groupings dip down into most communities with programs, resources, standards, requirements, expectations, rewards, and restrictions. They enlist help and support; they provide opportunities for affiliation and involvement; they make decisions that affect many aspects of life within the locality; and in a myriad of ways they exert direct and indirect influence. While such vertical associations also are affected by decisions and change at the local level, it usually is more difficult for local residents to recognize the influence they themselves may exert on national groups.

Virtually all organizations linking localities to state and national government and nongovernmental bodies are multilayered. From the local vantage point, authority and power reside "up the line." Influence and pressure seem to flow down far more easily than up. Such perceptions of discrepant power reflect the partial realities to be found in most situations. To an extent, however, they contribute to the reality itself, for they represent self-fulfilling prophecies. If the preponderance of power and authority is perceived to be up the line, those below may be hesitant to express concern or dissatisfaction openly and directly. Communications then become selective. Opinions and information that those in a position of responsibility might consider highly relevant, and which might cause a change in policy or action, are never received. Meanwhile, dissatisfaction mounts and counterpressures build up, which in the end may produce delay or even abandonment of a program.

Kramer (1967), describing a successful effort to form a tenants' association at a Boston public housing project, makes the point that tenants can only become responsible and well-informed about health and related programs if they have the power and the right to negotiate and to grapple with details of organizing services for themselves and their children. He finds a persuasive parallel in the history of labor-management negotiations, whereby over many years the labor unions "gained necessary technical competence and sophistication to shape costly health and welfare policies" (p. 214).

Because of the problems of miscommunication, dissatisfaction, and program failure associated with the multilayered quality of the regional and national linkages, many workers in the community field prefer to encourage the initiation of change from the bottom up. Mental health planners, for example, have spoken of "getting to the grass roots." They hold up as a positive goal the enlistment of representatives of all levels of the community in mental health planning bodies, study committees, and boards of directors in mental health agencies. The role of the professional staff is to help the citizens determine which problems are to be tackled first and, given the selection of objectives, which procedures will be most effective in reaching them. True "bottom-up" problem solving implies the involvement of local citizenry from the initial phase of problem identification, through a sequence of appraisal, selection of action steps, and evaluation of the effort.

In point of fact, however, a considerable amount of "top-down" planning and initiation of change usually has occurred before any locality becomes involved in the change process. This is the case in mental health efforts as well as many other programs of community improvement. Legislative and administrative decisions within national agencies and governmental authorities determine which programs shall be made available to local communities. Large sums of money are directed toward certain purposes and not others. Pressures for change are intense at times; often they are completely outside the locality's sphere of influence.

Because of the rise of vertical systems of association and of the growing recourse to centralized planning at state and national levels, many of the change pressures with which communities are faced are on administrative, programmatic, and political considerations apart from the immediate consideration of local needs. In a few instances such change can be interposed via chains of command within vertical associations, as from a federal government agency to its local field office. Usually other sources of power and persuasion are necessary. A favored strategy, which maintains (theoretically at least) some degree of local autonomy and initiative, involves making available large sums of money for local use within defined problem areas (housing, economic development, mental health planning, etc.). Predetermined standards tend to define when, how, for what, and by whom money will be spent. Local groups are caught in the conflict created by the recognition that money is needed to help deal with the problem area, as against the concern over inability to control locally just how the money is to be used. Under the circumstances, few community groups refuse available funds. Communities compete for the funds. The pressure to secure them is so great that sometimes money is applied for and granted before the problem has been adequately defined and the various consequences of a particular action plan have been thought through.

An increasingly important function of the professional change agent in mental health may become that of helping local community groups anticipate the total effects for the ecology of the community of establishing a new program in a particular area. It also is possible to help local groups relate themselves more effectively to vertical power pyramids. The process of planned change is as applicable to vertical associations as it is to the horizontal associations of the locality. It is not easy to achieve, however.

CHANGE IS RECIPROCAL

In most instances the initiation of change and maintenance of initiative through the change process probably occur simultaneously from top-down and bottom-up. Even in the city described by Hunter (1953) in which certain decisions were made by a small elite of power figures, most community decisions and actions were made and taken without participation by the elite. The reciprocal interplay between top and bottom is reinforced by the fact that a growing number of local problems involve state and national governmental and other bodies.

A mental health worker enters a community at the request of a local group of citizens. From the standpoint of the state mental health authority that hires the worker, he is responding to an appeal from the bottom up. Once in the community, the worker may discover that the requesting group is itself at the top of the several hierarchies. He may then attempt to translate community action, which in effect has been from the top down, into an attempt to involve many segments of the community in a study of its mental health needs and resources. At this point, the process has shifted to a bottom-up approach. When finally the assessment of needs has been completed and the community requests state help in establishing a mental health center, there is a return, in part, to top-down influence as the state authorities communicate certain minimal regulations and standards governing their participation in and support of the local program.

Thus we can probably treat the question most realistically by thinking of it not in dichotomized terms of "top" versus "bottom," but rather as a matter of several processes falling at various points along a continuum. It is essential that there be awareness of this continuum and of a project's position on it at any step in the change process. The zeal for bottom-up problem solving may lead to the error of asking people at the grass roots to make decisions beyond their capabilities, knowledge of facts, and abilities to uncover such knowledge. Similarly, apathy or hostility to change may reflect a situation where clinging to top-down initiation blocks those most directly involved in a problem from participating in attempts to solve it. A rule of thumb successfully used in some

industrial and other organizations is that decisions be made at the levels
where relevant facts are available and where solutions will be implemented. In applying the rule, it is essential that inadequate knowledge
and incapacity not be confused. Inadequate knowledge can be overcome
if sufficient time is taken for needed communication and education.

A critical challenge facing today's complex society is to provide adequate means for communicating up the line from the local community
through the several major vertical pyramids to state and national levels.
As was mentioned earlier, it is only through such communication that
technical high-level planners will have crucial information without
which plans can be little more than technological abstractions devoid of
the human element. In order to maintain the necessary communication
channels, some sort of integrative arrangements are necessary at the local
level. Here the various interests and needs of local groups can be
brought together and considered in relation to one another. Here, too,
decisions can be made about those concerns which must be shared vertically if particular goals are to be accomplished. More will be said about
horizontal and vertical integration in Chapter Fifteen.

The answer to the question raised by the title of this chapter is that
community change must become more and more collaborative. Involvement of residents is becoming increasingly accepted by those responsible
for major new social programs. Citizen participation, many believe, is
not only an ethical imperative; it is also more efficient. Thus it is being
built into major government programs, such as those of the Office of
Economic Opportunity, Model Cities, and Comprehensive Health Planning. There are many problems associated with citizen participation,
such as who is to be considered a *bona fide* representative of citizens,
how are they to be selected, what are their constituencies, and what relationship will they have to duly elected public officials? Despite the problems, however, efforts to involve citizens persist if only because more and
more people, including the formerly inarticulate poor, become unwilling
to acquiesce passively to the interventions of planners, however expert
and dedicated they may be. Mental health workers have much to offer
toward efforts to involve citizens in planning. They are in a position to
help planners and public officials be more understanding of and deal
more effectively with the inevitable problems of trust, authority, apathy,
and hostility.

CHAPTER THIRTEEN

Social Roles in Innovation

THE INNOVATION CURVE

The problems and processes involved in the effort to introduce new practices in a community are strikingly similar, across a wide range of technical areas. Studies of these dynamics in the introduction of such changes as new farming methods or innovations in medical practice have been carried out. They highlight a regularly recurring pattern of change in the adoption of new approaches, the so-called "innovation curve."

Lippitt and his colleagues at the University of Michigan Center for Research on the Utilization of Scientific Knowledge point out that innovation in areas of social practice, by comparison with applied biological and physical science, are more apt to require "significant changes in the values, attitudes, and skills of the social practitioner." (Lippitt, 1965, p. 668)

Investigators have repeatedly found that there is change at the outset of virtually any process of innovation. An innovation is usually tried out first by an atypical member of the group, such as a high-prestige figure who can afford to run the social or economic risk of failure, or someone who is so economically marginal that he has nothing to lose. Such individuals rarely serve as leaders, however, for they are too atypical. There is the fear, moreover, that initial success was only a fluke. Those who are more typically situated economically, socially, or emotionally will still hold back. To be more widely adopted, therefore, the new practice must be *adapted* (i.e., taken over), frequently with modifications that integrate them better with previous practices, by those persons who are perceived by their fellows as more typical. If now successful, there usually follows a rapidly accelerating curve of acceptance, although a minority usually resists to the end. This innovation sequence or curve describes quite well what I have observed as communities have reacted to the introduction of mental health programs.

INFORMAL COMMUNITY–CHANGE ROLES

Members of groups and organizations, and citizens of communities, assume certain social roles when confronted with the possibility of change. These roles are highly relevant to the process of innovation. In fact it may be postulated that orderly and successful change could not take place without them. Although there are many variations and subtypes, five seem most typical and most critical to community change. They are (a) the innovators, (b) the experimenters, (c) the adapters, (d) the defenders, and (e) the facilitators. There is in addition the less active but usually essential category of the uninvolved whom Leys (1952) has called the "bystanders."

THE INNOVATORS

This term refers to those who, dissatisfied with an aspect of the status quo, determine to alter it through the introduction of some new approach or practice. They are often from outside the locality, or, if situated within the community, are cosmopolitan in orientation. Innovators frequently appeal to resources, ideas, experiences, and other supports outside the locale.

THE EXPERIMENTERS

This term is used to denote those in an especially favorable position to experiment with new practices. These are the citizens of high prestige whose social position cannot be diminished if the experiment fails, or whose economic security permits them to take risks not allowed ordinary people. They also may be the members of the community who, in a sense, have nothing to lose from failure since they are already marginal economically or socially.

THE ADAPTERS

Once an individual or organization who can afford the risk has demonstrated that a new practice worked for him, there is still the necessity to discover whether and how the procedure can be taken over by the ordinary, run-of-the-mill person or group. Special factors may have enabled the experimenter to be successful. Perhaps some modifications will be necessary before the method can be used economically, safely, and effectively by all concerned. The adapters are those who take over the procedure, usually with major modifications or often only in a partial sense, for more widespread adoption (e.g., though certain experimenters have tried out community-wide, pervasive preventive approaches in community mental health, the trend today is for certain practices only to be taken over in a partial sense within more traditionally oriented settings). Mental health consultation is one such technique that has been both experimented with and adapted for use within existing and more traditional mental health agencies.

THE DEFENDERS

As the term suggests, here are the individuals and groups who resist the innovation. If it proves to be inevitable, they fight it and seek to control or encapsulate it within some limited sphere. In the process they perform a highly useful social function (i.e., they act in order to protect existing beliefs and ways of doing things). They ensure stability and avoid wildcat experimentation with unproved practices that may later backfire. If defenders function effectively in the process of change and innovation, they will enhance the problem solving process by requiring careful examination of the disadvantages as well as advantages of what is proposed. In so doing they may illuminate alternative goals, significant values and issues that had been overlooked, or direct attention to possible solutions for problems heretofore not considered.

THE FACILITATORS

These are the ones who focus attention on orderly processes of problem solving. They emphasize commonality of interests and community identifications on the part of conflicting factions. They play the roles of mediators, fact finders, facilitators of communication and reality testers. These functions are, as was suggested earlier in the consideration of planned change, part of the role of the change agent, be he professional or citizen. However, facilitators may perform their functions without seeking to move a situation toward any particular goal, save that of finding a resolution of a problem.

THE BYSTANDERS

By remaining outside the circle of those engaged in struggle, the bystanders play an important part in the dynamic of community conflict, controversy, and change; for, though disengaged, they are spectators who may decide to exert influence in one of several ways. It is as if the spectators in the Roman circus could jump down into the arena and join in the struggle on the side of a favored gladiator, as well as exert the life-or-death giving prerogative of signaling thumbs up or down to indicate the fate of a defeated protagonist. The bystanders frequently are courted by the partisans in the hope of enlisting their support. Sometimes they enter controversy only when it threatens to impair fundamental community cohesiveness and damage some community function. On the international scene, as we know, the bystander role is significantly played by the so-called neutralist or uncommitted countries, which form a body of world opinion that, hopefully, restrains the warring factions. It is clear from the world scene that the role is a vital one. It is also clear that when conflict mounts there are many pressures moving bystanders to relinquish that role. Finally, it may be noted that the bystander role can affect all the others; it is far less passive than the term implies.

FACTORS AFFECTING CHANGE ROLES

What determines the adoption of one or another community-change role by an individual or group? Are there factors other than the obvious one of personality characteristics (e.g., the predilection of certain people always to be for or against, to be challenging and critical or supportive and facilitating)? I think there are. Among the determinants should be listed such things as the nature of the individual's group memberships, others' expectations of him, direct or indirect interpersonal pressures, as well as the relationship between the person's own goals or needs and his membership or commitment to group and community. Observations of face-to-face groups over time, for example, suggest that individuals develop reputations which shape their behavior within the group. These reputations are difficult to alter and often must be expressed by the group member in ways that would not be manifest outside the particular group context. As I have attended New England town meetings year after year, I have strengthened my conviction that individuals perpetuate informal change roles not out of personality alone, but also out of their embeddedness within the life of the community. Certain behaviors are expected from certain people; others respond to them in predictable ways and, in effect, elicit these behaviors from them. Some of the more conspicuous actors have their cliques who respond appreciatively and participate vicariously as their spokesmen hold forth.

If the community-change roles adopted by individuals are not entirely a function of personality, it follows that each individual may take more than one role on different occasions (e.g., the citizen innovator, in a move to establish compulsory driver education in the high schools, might conceivably be found as a defender against the introduction of fluorides into the town water supply). The reader possibly will recall instances in which he or she has performed each of the six roles discussed earlier.

Any one of the change roles may become rigid and therefore played out long past the point where it is valuable. In the case of the defender, for example, there are many psychic rewards to be derived from upholding eternal verities. It is difficult to persuade a defender to jeopardize his reputation as one of the trustworthy shields for the community. The problem is complicated by the fact that the motivations for assuming the defender role (or any of the others, for that matter) may include such factors as need for power, desire for enhancement of prestige, or avoidance of personal threat. It is sometimes difficult for an individual or group to see that the situation has changed to the point where a certain change role is no longer functional or appropriate.

In part such rigidity is maintained inadvertently by those who ascribe the individual's rigidity to defects of personality: "He's just stubborn," or defects in moral fiber: "All he cares about is power." Change may be made possible by applying the principle of providing a substitute defense for one that is threatened. What works in the psychotherapeutic process may also apply in a community situation that seems impervious to change. It may be possible, for example, for defenders to develop a sense of belonging to a new group in which roles are developed that are both personally enhancing and relatively free of personal threat. Such a development is likely if truly reciprocal relationships are maintained between the incumbents of the several informal change roles .(e.g., innovators may find themselves relying on the erstwhile defenders for indoctrination into the central beliefs and traditions of the community). Under such circumstances the defender will not cease playing this role. He will continue to defend his community by assuring that orderly change occurs and that problem solving efforts are based on the widest possible knowledge of the relevant facts and alternative solutions.

Some applied behavioral scientists (among them Lippitt and his group) have been particularly interested in identifying and devising ways in which behavioral science consultants, among whom hopefully will be many mental health workers, can facilitate both innovation and diffusion of social practices. Collaborative data gathering in the field as well as experimental field testing of new procedures are among the more traditional approaches they are using. In addition they are especially impressed by the potential for creative change that might be realized if ways were developed to identify and document imaginative and effective new practices that have already been tried out elsewhere. Lippitt points out that much social practice (e.g., in both education and mental health) remains "relatively invisible." The result is that there is little competitive challenge, stimulation to communicate what has been discovered, or desire to search out the innovations of others. Too much of what is both new and well grounded in research and theory does not become visible and "never becomes transmitted from one setting and practitioner to another, with the tragic outcome that high quality adoption is impossible" (Lippitt, 1965, p. 666).

Vigorous promotion of good social innovation and dissemination practices may be one of the most needed community functions that can be performed by mental health teams. The community mental health center itself may become a focal resource in the network of procedures and transmission points that are badly needed if social research is to be effectively linked to social practice. It can only do so, however, if its staff understands the innovation and dissemination process and is aware of its critical potential for participating in and fostering it.

CHAPTER FOURTEEN

Social Conflict and Community Change

THE NATURE OF CONFLICT

Until now I have barely distinguished between situations in which disagreements occur in a context of trust and collaboration and those involving mistrust, polarization of positions, and head-on conflict. The
force-field model would suggest that the extreme build-up of conflicting
forces results in a tension-filled, markedly unstable state. This model
also suggests that conflict involves the confrontation of individuals,
groups, or other aggregates that are seeking to achieve *mutually exclu-
sive goals*. It is not possible, for example, to both fluoridate the water
supply of a city and not to do so at one and the same time. For the situation to be truly conflicting, however, one further criterion must be met:
the achievement of its objectives by one party to the dispute must be
experienced by the other as loss or defeat. This is true, of course, in the
case of the fluoridation example. But there are many situations where
the achievement of one group's goals is not experienced by another
group as defeat of itself, even though the achievement in actuality may
limit the latter's chances of having its way. An example of such a situation was involved when the board of aldermen of a city decided to re-
model the central library, and later turned down plans for expansion of
the trade school because of lack of funds. The trade school protagonists,
pleased with the library decision, and not having defined the problem as
involving a choice in the allocation of limited funds, did not experience
the library victory as a defeat for their cause. True conflict involves
either the actual use of violence or at the very least a strong sense of
struggle among antagonists. It is accomplished by a tendency to polarize—to simplify issues into right and wrong, decisions into yes or no,

groups and individuals into for and against or good and bad. It is difficult, often impossible, to identify with or develop empathy for one's antagonists in a conflict situation. Concomitantly, there is a strengthening of loyalties and ties within each of the warring factions. Between opposing groups there is distrust. Often each group projects all that is bad onto the opposition.

A recent dispute was observed between a student group and a business concern that the students accused of racial discrimination in its hiring practices. The personnel director presented the students with facts about the proportion of Negroes in its work force and the rate of new hirings among black and white applicants. The students insisted that the progress reported by the company was not enough. As discussion proceeded, it was clear that student distrust was so great that virtually nothing the company representatives could suggest would be satisfactory. Later interviews revealed that the students did not trust the company, would not accept the facts presented by the representatives, and could not conceive of a proposition from the company that would be satisfactory.

The preceding example highlights another characteristic of many conflict situations: they tend to be self-perpetuating because of the climate of distrust and the commitment to engage in the struggle until the opposition is overcome. Communication becomes virtually impossible in such circumstances. Almost all messages from one side to the other become distorted by the opposition as they are viewed as further evidences of why "we" cannot trust "them."

THE NATURAL HISTORY OF COMMUNITY CONFLICT

The phenomena that result in conflict in communities are well described by Coleman (1959) in his reconstruction of the "natural history" of a number of such situations. He suggests that previously suppressed hostilities between opponents must be present for any particular issue to serve as the vehicle for conflict. As a specific issue enters the picture and begins to affect community equilibrium, underlying cleavages bob to the surface. The focus shifts inexorably from a disagreement over issues to an open fight between sides. Each stereotypes the other as inherently evil, unprincipled, or at the very least, misguided. Coleman also notes that such disputes tend to become independent of the initial issue. As events develop, the issues change from specific to general disagreements; disagreement becomes direct antagonism; and in the ultimate conflict situation, the community itself becomes split into warring camps.

THE VALUE OF CONFLICT

Do the foregoing observations about change and conflict lead to the conclusion that conflict is to be avoided whenever possible? What are the implications for those concerned with community mental health? Certainly in the mental health approach there is an implicit value attached to the reduction of conflict and the management of conflict through rational means. Emotional well-being could hardly be expected to thrive in a conflict-laden social environment.

Yet, it may be argued that in community situations, as in the life of the individual, conflict cannot always be avoided; when necessary it should be accepted and utilized as part of the social change process (Benne, undated). Certainly, mental health principles would suggest that where conflict exists, it is preferable to confront it directly rather than to suppress it or deny its existence.

There are those who, far from believing that conflict should be avoided whenever possible, hold that conflict should never be avoided unless absolutely necessary. Some believe that delay in bringing potential contention to the conflict level simply plays into the hands of those seeking to maintain the status quo. Saul Alinsky (1946, 1965) is the best known, but by no means the only, authority holding to this viewpoint. These workers maintain that major changes cannot be achieved without conflict. They view conflict as a desirable means for highlighting the existence of problems, for emphasizing the urgency of a situation, for creating solidarity within the groups fighting for change, and for energizing previously unconcerned or apathetic individuals who under ordinary circumstances play little part in community life (Kerr, 1954; Coser, 1956; Hallenback, 1960). Coser especially emphasizes that conflict satisfies some of man's more primitive needs, which have few if any outlets in modern society. When caught up in fighting for a cause greater than themselves alone, many individuals are enabled to vent long-smouldering frustrations. There is no doubt in my mind that conflict is a necessary and not simply an inevitable part of living, whether seen on the internal or external, on the biologic or interpersonal, on the community or larger societal levels. If this is true, it follows that a viable community must contain within it some suitable and nondestructive means for allowing conflict to occur. Mumford (1938) has suggested that many utopian communities have failed in their purposes because they sought on idealistic grounds to rule out conflict rather than to embody suitable means for confronting and dealing with it.

Differences in attitude toward the desirability and inevitability of conflict in the modern community stem partly from semantic confusion. Some use the term "conflict" to denote increased tension, while others use it to denote extreme crisis; some are concerned with differences over goals to be sought, while others restrict themselves to the existence of actual contention between factions.

SOURCES OF CONFLICT

Whether we define it as increased tension or open controversy, conflict cannot be avoided by the mental health team. At one time or another the mental health movement will find itself caught up in community conflicts which can spring from any one of a number of sources. Various lists of the sources of community conflict have been drawn up (e.g., Coleman, 1959; Nelson et al., 1960; Hallenback, 1960). Without attempting to be exhaustive, the following paragraphs take up a few of them as they might affect mental health programs.

Possibly most fundamental are those differences in backgrounds, beliefs, and values which are to be found among the residents of almost all modern communities of any size. Religious beliefs, for example, are a potent source of division. They influence voting behavior, shape stands on social issues, determine attitudes toward international affairs, not to mention their influence on the extent to which individuals support and patronize mental health facilities. Certain religious groups are more heavily represented than others among the professional and citizens groups devoted to the extension of mental health programs. Other groups believe that religious and mental health values are fundamentally and irreconcilably opposed. All of this simply underscores the fact that the mental health field itself is a social movement, embodying an identifiable set of values, and competing in the market place for the interest, loyalty, and support of the citizens. In the process mental health must come into conflict with other movements whose values are, or appear to be, in opposition to those that it espouses.

Related to value concerns are such matters as age, education, and mobility. It is apparent that mental health has been more congenial to the younger, more highly educated, and often more mobile segments of our communities. Older people, those without college education, and those whose roots in their communities go back for generations, have been less likely to become enthusiastic supporters of recent developments in comprehensive mental health. There is a ready source of conflict here between mental health supporters and their opponents, especially since very often the initial impetus for the development of mental health facilities comes from a relative newcomer to a community or even from an outside group brought in specifically for the purpose of promoting the mental health cause.

As we have seen, there are in most of our large communities today large numbers of people, often the impoverished, ethnic minorities, but by no means only them, who feel isolated, alienated, and cut off from the centers of power. The middle-class supporters of mental health centers rarely are to be found among these disenfranchised groups. They come mainly from the ranks of the joiners—the relatively small minority of people who become active members and leaders of the many groups and organizations concerned with the business, health, welfare, and other facets of community life. Those who feel outside the spheres of power can readily distrust and therefore oppose the development of mental health resources that they have not helped to shape and that they may view as still another activity devoted to exposing their inadequacies.

The political process, too, may be a potent source of conflict when it comes to mental health matters and other issues of civic improvement. Who, for example, is to decide whether to establish a mental health program? Which individuals will determine what groups are to be served and what services are to be offered them? In recent years there has been in some states an eruption of conflict between citizens' mental health associations, traditionally active in the field, and governmental authorities, more recently taking on responsibilities for community-centered programs. The locus of power and influence in mental health has shifted rapidly from the citizens' group to governmental bodies. To what extent, if at all, will citizens in the future share in policy making and direction setting for the government financed mental health centers? Such questions have more than casual interest to those who recognize that the careers of political figures and the success of political campaigns may rest on how adequately the mental health job is done. They have at least as much interest to those who sense that the growing community mental health "industry" will of necessity involve the expenditure of large sums and a substantial increase in employment opportunities for semiskilled as well as professional people in areas where programs are located.

Commenting on the inevitability of conflict, Nelson (1959) has pointed up the seemingly inherent capacity of man to misperceive and, therefore, distrust the motives of others. He writes, "Conflict . . . is at the very heart of life, resulting not simply from the malevolence of others in the struggle for place or portion, but also from the fact that men of the best will in the world seem to suffer incurably, so far as one can tell, from what William James called 'a certain blindness' in perceiving the vitalities of others" (p. 147).

MANAGEMENT OF CONFLICT

Though disagreement and contention are inevitable, even desirable, they can become destructive to the community. Constructive community action rarely results from extreme and sustained polarization. Locked-in and intense conflict situations in and of themselves lead neither to trust nor community cohesion among those who have been in contention. It is important, therefore, to search for ways in which conflicts can be handled effectively and creatively before they result in reduced community integration. Several models have been suggested.

We have already spent some time on Lewin's model of equilibrium and force field, which presents one approach to the understanding of conflict and its resolution (Lewin, 1958). The obvious strategy is to seek for ways to reduce the total tension on both sides of the equilibrium by removing or dampening the strength of the forces arrayed pro and con.

One of the earliest conflict resolution models was presented by Stuart Chase (1951), who proposed four principles as the basis for reaching agreements. Most of these have been discussed already in this volume in other contexts. They are:

1. Participation—the involvement of various members and segments of the community in the process of seeking agreement;

2. The mobilization of group energy through providing ways and means for action to be taken in the search for facts and possible solutions;

3. Communication—the fullest possible use of the mass media and the total array of techniques available for conveying attitudes and information to all concerned;

4. Confidence—encouragement of the feeling that solutions are possible and that, given sufficient effort and wisdom, action can and will be taken.

From the psychotherapeutic model of change can be derived the postulate that conflicts will be resolved only when people can be helped to perceive their true nature and origins. In the process of making known the true nature of the conflict the therapist usually must help the individual to deal with intrapsychic resistances which tend to subvert attempts to move toward more mature resolutions. He knows that when a defense against some unconscious impulse is weakened or set aside, there is an increase in anxiety and tension. These feelings will become overwhelming unless other mechanisms are developed for expressing and controlling the impulses. This therapeutic principle is applied to community conflict by the Mials (1960), who underscore the need to help the community diagnose and make visible the true nature and sources of the conflict. The Mials add that those working with conflicting groups should help them search for and identify overlapping objectives which they hold in common. Though sometimes of only low priority in any one group's goal hierarchies, such overlap does provide a common ground on which conflict-free interaction may be established. Sometimes the common goal simply may be a shared interest in the welfare of the community itself and a concern lest prolonged conflict might weaken it seriously.

Radical models of conflict management and social change do not seek to resolve conflict, but rather to promote and use it. The Hegelian theory is an example. Oversimplifying Hegel's postulates, this model builds on an acceptance of the inevitability of conflict. It postulates that new resolutions or syntheses emerge from each conflictual upheaval. Each emergence is opposed in its turn. This leads to new conflict, and the ultimate emergence of new synthesis, and so on. In Lewin's terms, the Hegelian orientation that one should seek change by promoting conflict, means that one should add to driving forces in an effort to overcome all opposition.

A somewhat similar position is held by those who seek to bring about social change by legal means (i.e., by adding legal pressures to the driving forces already working toward a desired end). Among these people is Louis Wirth (1956), who believes that the use of legal means is both rapid and effective, in contrast to other more gradual approaches, just because it sharpens the conflict most forcefully for all concerned. The conflict becomes one between law and social custom. If people's traditions also encompass obedience to law, there results a set of sharply contrasting and incompatible norms, to both of which people subscribe.

It is at least as valid to view law as the manifestation of a complex process of social change and conflict resolution that is already taking place. The ability of a segment of society to initiate change in law reflects (a) the prevailing pattern of sentiments and (b) differential patterns of access to law making and law interpreting institutions enjoyed by different segments of the society. Prestige groups and others through high socioeconomic status, accepted leadership, and friendship, may influence law even though they are in the minority. Or, highly organized and articulate groups may coalesce successfully around clearly defined issues that they feel touch them personally. Excellent examples of the latter are to be found in the highly effective efforts of many antifluoridation groups in local communities, and of parents of retarded children who have succeeded in having passed special legislation to meet the needs of their children and others like them.

Another approach to conflict management is based on analysis of the communication patterns and processes. As we have already seen, massive barriers often block exchange of information even in the simplest of interpersonal and intergroup situations. Difficulties in achieving change often compound problems. Breakdown in communication is seen as leading to serious conflict. The resolution of the conflict rests on establishment of communication. Efforts to improve communication when successful may lead to a new and more differentiated perception of the problem. Groups previously in conflict with one another may, with improved communication, perceive that differences are not irreconcilable and that, indeed, they share the common goal of wishing to benefit the community.

Communication is facilitated when those involved are helped to develop a sense of shared identifications. Mead (1934) put the problem in terms of the ability to take the role of the other. Others have suggested that propinquity and opportunities for contact under benign circumstances may help develop such intergroup empathy. It is recognized that communication by itself is no panacea. Conflicts may be reality based, and communication will only underscore this fact. As one group opens its eyes to what the other group has been feeling all along, there may be temporary increases in conflicts (e.g., the current hostile white reactions to Negro activist groups and proponents of black power). Finally, it may well be that breakdown in communication is at times functional for the community, just as in the individual defenses are erected to ward off the direct expression or even consciousness of unacceptable impulses.

The basic assumption underlying the communication approach to conflict resolution is derived from psychotherapeutic experience and intergroup experiences in the religious, racial, and industrial fields. It holds that mutual exploration by the factions of previously uncharted depths leads to rational understanding of the nature of the problem; that with increased understanding comes better organization of controls, more effective channels of communication, and therefore more opportunities to secure relevant information, leading in the end to the institution of better patterns for solving future problems.

CHAPTER FIFTEEN

Integrative Patterns in Community Life

Patterns of integration refer to the ways in which individuals relate to one another and to the community as well as to the ways in which resources are coordinated for the common good. In many communities today patterns of integration are shifting as old ways prove inadequate and new ways emerge which challenge existing structures. The new patterns often are confusing to, and even bitterly opposed by, established leaders and many of their constituents. Once again it is the story of accelerating technological change, rapid population growth, the mobility of many citizens (including some of the groups from which community leadership typically is drawn), and the creation of larger and even more complex political and functional jurisdictions to cope with health, education, transportation, and other needs.

Despite turbulent currents of change and conflict, however, most communities manage to avoid major disruptions. They do so through integrative forces that are poorly understood and deserve far more study than they have so far received. Though these forces are unclear and harder to grasp than processes of change, conflict, or disruption, they are as essential to community life and as fundamental to an understanding of community as are ego structure and coping mechanisms to an understanding of personality. The assessment of any community's dynamics is grossly incomplete if it leaves out the patterns and processes whereby (a) individuals become related to one another through informal associations and formal organizations, (b) individuals, groups, and organizations interact in order to deal with recurring problems and meet new challenges, and (c) the community copes with the growing demands from the world outside its geographic boundaries.

INTEGRATING THE INDIVIDUAL

Certain value considerations must be faced at the outset. I do not believe that the broad interests of mental health will be served by a future society that resembles Huxley's *Brave New World,* in which the great mass of humanity is conditioned to function without choice as an unthinking proletariat. To the contrary, I believe it is more consistent with good mental health for people to have opportunities to cope actively with their environment and to influence it for good or ill. It is good mental health for people to be able to use to the fullest their intellectual and emotional capabilities for the welfare of others as well as themselves. It is good mental health for people to be valued members of the community and to know that they may be included within and accepted by social groupings important to them.

There is no doubt that failure in integration profoundly affects the rate and nature of use of the cultural, economic, and helping resources of the community. We have long known that certain multiproblem families were parceled out among a host of agencies unrelated to one another (Buell, 1952). More recently we have clear evidence that the poor typically have less access than other economic groups to basic welfare, educational, and health (mental as well as physical) resources (Riessman and Scribner, 1965; Miller, 1965).

Leaving aside the matter of resource utilization, many people fail to establish the semblance of participation in community life in those respects that build significance and basic security. They suffer from the agonizing anonymity of the perpetual stranger. Or they are oppressed by the sense of worthlessness and futility arising from inability to influence the course of events.

The plight of such marginal men in our midst has been a matter of increasing concern to mental health and other experts. Some promising beginning efforts are underway and are designed to connect marginal individuals with the mainstream of society (e.g., Daniels' and Koldau's program of providing a patient-managed employment service in a Veterans Administration Hospital (1967) and the well known Synanon program for rehabilitation of drug addicts described by Yablonski, 1965).

The Negro who cannot register to vote is not the only one who feels himself disenfranchised; nor is it only the urban poor who feel marginal, alienated, or powerless. There are many others who feel cut off from the sources of community power. Their spokesmen, when they exist, are not part of the establishment. Thus their thinking is apt to be dismissed by those in power as unsound, and community action proceeds with neither their understanding nor their consent. It is only when issues become simplified and reduced to the most concrete choice between accepting or rejecting a specific course of action that those who feel powerless may rise up against the powers that be. Viewed in this way, the fluoridation controversy becomes as much a symptom of disenfranchisement as it is a health issue. The method of referendum itself ensures the average citizen a voice in community affairs when he feels cut off from or betrayed by those who purport to represent him.

Integration of the individual within community life occurs in many ways other than through political action. The arena for participation may be as restricted as when kinsmen live within easy walking, riding, perhaps telephoning distance, or as limited as the block or neighborhood where one dwells. The arena for some is the single community. These individuals are the "locals," so called because their primary identifications and associations are with fellow residents of the local geographic community. Others seek to integrate within several communities. If they are unsuccessful, there is conflict; the individual is torn between seemingly irreconcilable demands. The resulting loss affects both the person and the communities. If successful, they may achieve a kind of harmonious cosmopolitanism in which multiple citizenships within professional, recreational, political, and cultural groupings are cemented together by a core of common values shared with fellow cosmopolitans. Lowry (1965, p. 144) has invented the term "mediating leader" to refer to an individual who, in his words, "maintains overlapping memberships and informal relationships with both local and cosmopolitan groups." Lowry's studies suggest that mediating leaders are drawn from diverse fields, all of which have in common the fact that their occupational roots are in both the locality and the larger society.

Certain bedroom communities surrounding large urban centers suffer from the multiple community memberships of their residents. Affairs of the locality are left in the hands of a few store owners, town employees, and others who live and work there. One community's remedy in the greater Boston area was the formation of an organization of commuting business executives and professional men, which met monthly to discuss matters affecting their suburb. By meeting in Boston during the day it was possible to enlist the interest and participation of many who could not be drawn into town affairs through evening meetings after a long working day.

Some locals and many cosmopolitans establish integration with the community through organizational memberships. Many reflect the variety of subcommunities which cluster around ethnic, social class, religious, political, professional, business, labor, and other common characteristics. It is within these groupings that values are developed, reinforced, or altered; common identities are formed and maintained; political and social attitudes are shaped and hardened. In one sense such organizations reflect the most prevalent cleavages among segments of a community. Participation within one such subcommunity tends to rule out contact and communication with another. In another sense, however, these groupings become the platforms from which intergroup collaboration, planning, and problem-solving become possible if there are mechanisms for interorganizational contact.

The community participation of an individual is partly shaped by his personality and past experience, but it also is strongly influenced by his milieu. Whyte's study of Park Forest, Illinois (1956) revealed that quite different patterns of community participation emerged in otherwise similar neighborhoods. In one section, for example, there was much neighboring and sharing of recreational interests, but little interest in overall community issues. In another section, inhabited more or less randomly by people having socioeconomic characteristics comparable to those of the other sections, there was little partying but deep involvement in civic affairs and political action.

Observations of the adjustment of newcomers were made by the mental health program in Wellesley (Thoma and Lindemann, 1961). The quality and nature of the adaptation appeared to depend on three factors: (a) the skill demonstrated by family members in relating to new people and customs, (b) the readiness of the neighborhood to reach out to newcomers, and (c) the extent to which existing organizations and institutions corresponded to previous membership experiences of the family. Newcomers' clubs and such commercial welcoming organizations as Welcome Wagon also played a part. In one tract of new homes grateful wives held a cocktail party in honor of an especially friendly and knowledgeable Welcome Wagon lady who had helped them make the transition to the community.

COORDINATION WITHIN THE COMMUNITY

At another level, community integration is the ability of citizens to enter into trustful relationships in order to assess and cope with common problems. The mechanisms vary—they include all the official elected and appointed bodies of government; supervisory, administrative, and planning boards and committees; formally established councils of health and welfare; voluntary fund-raising and allocating groups; and *ad hoc* coalitions in specific problem areas, such as mental health or smoking control; professional associations; informal groups and clusters of opinion leaders; service clubs; and such nonpartisan study and education organizations as the League of Women Voters. They employ almost all conceivable means for communication and influence: face-to-face contact; radio, newspaper, and television; pamphlets and flyers; and in some instances, even highly effective telephone networks capable of mobilizing sentiment and action in a matter of hours.

The basic dynamics of community integration which underlie observable structures and mechanisms usually cannot be observed directly. Nevertheless, the astute observer can develop a feeling for them as he talks with inhabitants, and asks himself such questions as:

1. To what extent do people have a sense of common destiny within this locality; what kind of community identity, if any, do they have in common?

2. Is community leadership available that seems adequate to cope with the demands of the situation?

3. Is there a sense of mutual respect and trust between groups of citizens and between citizens and their leaders?

4. What kind of reputation do residents think their community has among outsiders?

High integration is reflected by a shared sense that there is a positively valued common destiny which binds people together. Opportunities for participation in community affairs are felt to exist for all levels and segments of the population. Residents know that it is possible for groups to put aside differences in order to cope with overriding problems. There is a sense of self-worth that is reflected in the belief that outsiders view the community and its inhabitants positively.

Leighton and his co-workers (Hughes et al., 1960) have identified seven preliminary indicators of community disintegration that can be noted without extensive interviewing or detailed study of records. They are:

1. A recent history of economic or other disaster affecting the basic means of livelihood;

2. Widespread ill health;

3. Extensive poverty;

4. A confusion of cultural backgrounds in which little or no synthesis of differing culture values is occuring;

5. Weakening of membership in religious groups with consequent secularization of the inhabitants;

6. Extensive migration of new groups;

7. Rapid social change affecting many of the traditional patterns of community life.

In their studies of several Nova Scotian towns the Leighton group found that communities high in the seven preliminary indicators also were likely to show serious symptoms of social pathology in several spheres. In a disintegrated town weakening of primary group ties resulted in a relatively high frequency of broken homes. Residents claimed few friendships or other close associations. Communication between individuals and groups was infrequent and incomplete, and indeed, poor interpersonal relations were reflected in a high frequency of hostile expressions and behaviors. Recreational opportunities were sparse. Crime and juvenile delinquency were high. And it was clear that the few people in leadership positions were unable to exert strong authority or to mobilize community problem solving efforts. One indication of the Leighton findings is that community integration is highly vulnerable to disruption through the withdrawal of the economic base that provides employment, fiscal stability, and self-respect for the majority of wage earners and their families. Without this base morale breaks down, and minor cleavages become the basis for miscommunication and distrust. Often the most able, vigorous people move out, and those remaining find themselves trapped in a downward spiral of worsening disorganization. In such situations mental health problems such as delinquency cannot be approached apart from an attack on the more basic conditions which have led to the disintegration. These principles form the basis for the community development approach which seeks to foster rediscovery of leadership potential and cohesiveness through self-help (Biddle and Biddle, 1965; Franklin, 1966).

COORDINATIVE COUNCILS

As public and private agencies concerned with health and welfare have multiplied in most communities, more and more distinct professional groups have joined in the attack on social and health problems. There has been an obvious need for coordination and planning, if only to reduce overlap in services and allocate limited resources for the greatest good. Multiple-problem families could not be served adequately if their many economic, health, and social difficulties were to be parceled out among agencies that were not acquainted with one another's work. Pressures toward coordinated community services came also from those whose charitable and tax dollars paid the bills. Professionals themselves agreed that coordination and planning might help to establish more adequate services and suitably high standards. It also was hoped that a coalition or federation of those most deeply committed to public health and welfare would result in more effective political action and better social legislation.

In communities all over the country charitable federation and health and welfare councils were formed. They took many forms, set differing objectives, placed greater or lesser emphasis upon lay or professional participation and control, and met with success, depending on the nature and extent of community sanction for their existence, adequacy or leadership, and many other factors. In recent years it has become clear that federated integration of local agencies has certain inherent difficulties. Some of them are especially weighty for those running community mental health programs. The typical community agency is concerned with a relatively narrow band of functions requiring specialized skills. The community council facilitates communication between them. When effective it is in a position to see that no agency infringes on the domain of another. Coordination becomes a matter of rationally deploying the specialized functions so that those in need will be able to call on appropriate services.

While the traditional mental hygiene clinic is readily integrated within such a complex of autonomous specialized resources, the more comprehensive mental health center is not. It seeks to offer generalized consulting services and wishes to enlist the collaboration of the specialized agencies in a comprehensive approach to prevention, care, and rehabilitation. In fact, the mental health program itself can become an integrative vehicle for other community agencies helping to bring them together for a concerted effort at bringing help to families and even entire neighborhoods in high need areas. An example is the Elm Haven Concerted Services Program of New Haven in which the Psychiatric Council is "the one unit (among at least ten concerned with health, education, employment, and other needs in a low-cost housing project) that operates in a horizontal fashion," by virtue of the fact that it is a consultant to all (Solnit, 1967, p. 505).

Though such programmatic integration is probably effective in the shortrun, it is doubtful that mental health units are acceptable to other agencies in the longrun as integrators of the social improvement efforts of a community. Perhaps there is a need for mechanisms whereby fluctuating short-term coalitions, such as Solnit describes, can be formed within the framework of more regularized means for community coordination, such as the interagency council.

In fact, however, the mechanism of the council often fails to deliver the kind of planned integration for which it was designed. Individual agencies and programs have strong support from different segments of the community. There is resistance to any council that seeks to move far beyond a communicative and coordinative function into a position of directing and controlling agency activities. In the face of vested interests even Community Chests, United Funds, and other coordinated voluntary fund-raising groups often have little power to redeploy financial support in major ways (Sanders, 1958).

The history of coordinative efforts at the community level within the United States is marked by a long string of brave and enthusiastic attempts, none of which have achieved the success hoped for by their protagonists. The community organization field in social work is noted for imaginative efforts to bring together professional workers and agency board leaders in a variety of health, welfare, and recreational councils. The community development field emerged in the early twentieth century with vigorous attempts to develop across-the-board participation of all segments of communities in programs of community improvement. These efforts continue today and are even entering a renaissance period, after a twenty year period in which community development appeared to be primarily for export to underdeveloped countries only (Mial, 1958).

The most recent and familiar examples of new attempts at coordinated efforts to bring about the rational redeployment of resources to meet complex problems, are the antipoverty programs of the Office of Economic Opportunity, the Model Cities planning efforts under the coordination of the Department of Housing and Urban Development, and the pilot neighborhood service center program.

All these efforts to integrate both horizontally and vertically the agencies and citizen groups—whether in the interest of efficiency, of more effective delivery and utilization of professional services for those in greatest need, or of a concerted attack on underlying causes of multiple social problems—have been marked by high hopes and, to an unfortunate extent, by the apparent conviction that previous efforts either never existed or were flawed by lack of will, ineptitude, or inadequate grasp of the real task (flaws that can somehow be avoided by the newest group to try).

No single rational system for planning and packaging human resources to meet the complex problems of today's community will succeed. It is likely that multiple packages for limited purposes will be required, such as the ones that mental health teams are developing with the cooperation of other groups. I hope that mental health efforts to build integrative mechanisms will be based on modest, attainable goals, and that they will avoid the trap of attempting to become the new forge on which the fully integrated community can be hammered out. Most of all, it is important to build on rather than to reject previous attempts, many of which are highly imaginative and at least partially successful, all of which provide techniques and insights that can be invaluable.

Some of the problems with which the comprehensive mental health center is concerned also involve the interests and competencies of other groups (e.g., mental retardation is also within the sphere of education, vocational rehabilitation, recreation, and medicine, to name just a few). Who is to take prime responsibility for coordination here? Can such a problem as mental retardation be handled completely within most existing community health and welfare councils? The answers are not yet clear. It is obvious, however, that new and frequently *ad hoc* coalitions are being formed in an attempt to deal with such broad problem areas by means of temporary task forces. Often they must encompass governmental agencies such as public education and public mental health authorities which have not usually been included within traditional community councils.

It is especially difficult for a council of community agencies to integrate the activities of voluntary agencies with government bodies. Voluntary agencies can be controlled if necessary through the council's ability either to allocate the charitable dollar or to exert influence upon its allocation. The fiscal and programmatic control of governmental authorities, however, must be in the hands of elected or appointed boards, which in turn usually are responsible to the mayor or other administrative heads of the government. Governmental agencies are subject to legal requirements and restrictions that make it difficult for them either to offer services that are adequate in the eyes of the voluntary agencies or to modify programs in keeping with the plans of a council. Among areas affected have been community health programs, usually under government auspices and often, therefore, not readily integrated with the work of the voluntary family, child care, and other social agencies. Mental health is increasingly being sponsored and financed by government. Because of this, it, too, is becoming less easily integrated within traditional health and welfare council patterns.

INTEGRATION BETWEEN
GOVERNMENTAL AUTHORITIES

From a superficial view, there should be few if any difficulties in integrating local public health, welfare, and educational programs. Administratively, they all appear to be part of the same city, town, or county government; the locus of coordinative responsibility must be in the administrative heads of that government, be they mayor, manager, selectmen, city council, or board of supervisors. Decisions can be made by a few people and presumably can be enforced by the allocation of the tax dollar and the power to command the loyalty of key subordinates.

Things simply do not work that way; governmental districts for health, welfare, educational, and other services often are not coterminous. Officials responsible for planning and implementation of health services may be under the aegis of county government; those responsible for welfare under the city or town; those responsible for education completely independent of either city or county officialdom.

The importance of the interagency integrative problem within the mental health field itself is reflected in a nationwide inquiry into school-related mental health programs conducted a few years ago (Hollister, 1963). It found that many local school systems' mental health programs had little or no contact, let alone collaboration, with local community mental health colleagues and programs. There was repeated fragmentation of services to children with emotional problems, based more on the nature of the symptoms than the underlying problems themselves. Thus a child with emotional stress at home might be a case for the attendance officer or school social worker if he truants, for the vice principal if he fights on the playground, for the school psychologist if his learning suffers, or the school nurse if he presents stomachaches or other physical symptoms.

Moreover, it was clear that no one was certain where the dividing line was, if any, between the schools' and the outside community's responsibilities for the care of children with moderate to severe emotional problems. There is no indication that the integrative dilemmas have been resolved in the several years since Hollister made his observations.

As if this were not enough, there has tended to be little attempt in some localities to establish any but the most casual communication or coordination between the separate domains, even when they are under the same governmental aegis. Outstanding exceptions do exist (e.g., coordinated health services may help plan and staff comprehensive health programs within public schools). Resistance to coordinated planning and programming sometimes comes from administrators who find that it is more difficult to direct and control personnel who cannot be hired and fired. At least as formidable an obstacle is the fact that often the several agencies must, in effect, compete for the allocation of tax revenues; it is usually easier to demonstrate a need for adding to an agency's direct specialized services than it is to justify the expenditure of public funds for committee meetings and other coordinative activities.

COPING WITH OUTSIDE FORCES: VERTICAL INTEGRATION

Local community coordination is caught in a rapidly worsening crossfire brought on partly by massive state and federal thrusts into major problem areas. Mental health is one such area, together with urban renewal, antipoverty programs, delinquency control, mental retardation, services for the elderly, and so on through virtually the entire gamut of our current social problems. These national groups are increasing their efforts to upgrade the work of local units through establishment of standards, education of professional and volunteer workers, and provision of regional consultants and troubleshooters. Sometimes, as was recently the case with the Girl Scouts of America, they have sought to integrate local community units into regional structures designed to ensure high caliber programs locally and to provide scarce staff consulting resources more readily to local groups. Still further turbulence is created by the rapid growth of metropolitan concentrations of populations for which intercommunity planning is an obvious necessity. Traditional coordinative structures are no longer adequate for the task of coping with the integration of so many powerful forces from the outside. Moreover, inadequate coordination at higher (i.e., national) levels among the agencies pushing the several programs creates serious discontinuities in planning, program development, and direct service at the local level (Bindman, 1966).

It is no doubt true, although some would deny it, that thrusts from the outside have resulted from the inability of local bodies to finance, coordinate, and staff adequate programs for the reduction or elimination of major social ills. Horizontal coordination within the single community has tended to maintain the existence of separate agencies whose total effect has been rather more ameliorative than preventive. There is, of course, little evidence yet that massive state or federal programs in the mental health or any other field will succeed any better in attacking the social and cultural roots of the malaise.

In any event, local communities are faced with the problem of integrating vertically as well as horizontally (Warren, 1956). Means must be found to ensure the realization of local values and the strengthening of local resources as vertically oriented programs impinge on the community. Otherwise, there can only be an increasing alienation of function "through the removal of the operational control of a function from the community it is supposed to serve" (Brownell, 1950, p. 15). The same alienation of the function of education and socialization, which occurred in hundreds of rural communities as a result of consolidated education, appears to have occurred in the urban village's relationship to the large, bureaucratized school system. Similar alienation occurs in other functions, among them health. Some efforts to redress the situation in education are being made by decentralizing school administration and creating local area citizen boards in such cities as New York. Storefront mental health centers and multiservice neighborhood centers are all part of a national trend to reduce the powerlessness of local groups in respect to critical areas of their lives.

The problem is almost overwhelming in magnitude and complexity. Most vertical programs, including those of mental health, lay claim on the time and energies of existing agencies and political leaders. Most seek to involve citizen groups in order to ensure acceptance of their programs and, in fact, some are required by law to do so. The result is that citizen leadership becomes diverted from existing local resources, however. There also is some question as to just how many simultaneous attacks on major social ills any community can survive, let alone handle adequately.

In some instances local agencies face the prospect of competing with one another for state or federal funds as new appropriations become available. If they choose not to do so, they must be prepared to face the formation of new units having relatively larger sums of money to spend, more highly paid staffs, and sometimes a more glamorous appeal to citizen leaders, especially those who find it satisfying to shift from a local to a cosmopolitan outlook. Once they receive outside money, local groups often find themselves in the position of having to conform with restrictions and guidelines as well as statements of program priority which have the effect of shaping purpose and activity apart from any assessment of local needs, traditions, attitudes, or ways of working. It is clear that the issues of local autonomy, states rights, and federal control are of great relevance to mental health operations.

The matter of vertical integration cuts both ways. Those in state, regional, or national positions must depend on local support for the smooth and effective implementation of programs. At the very least, local opposition to a program must be neutralized; agreement of key individuals and groups must be secured. At the very most, it is likely that local people, once their interests and energies are engaged, will be able to suggest program modifications, point up new needs, and otherwise help to shape more realistic goals and more effective attempts to achieve them.

Vertical integration takes place in various ways. Traditionally, of course, the major way in our democracy has been through the clashing and accommodation of local and regional interests in representative legislatures. Political parties, too, weld their national machineries in order to coalesce local and state, as well as national, interests and objectives. In so doing they ensure a degree of effective communication up as well as down the ladder and make it possible for local needs to be taken into account when regional and national decisions are made.

REGIONAL MECHANISMS

The United States Government has evolved a far-reaching regional office mechanism that seeks to act as a link between state health, education, and welfare authorities and the federal government. Consultants from regional offices work with state programs and see to it that federal requirements are met when federally financed programs are administered by states. In turn, they help convey local needs to appropriate sections of the United States Public Health Service and to other divisions within the Department of Health, Education, and Welfare.

The regional office mechanism is widely used by other Federal Departments and national voluntary agencies. This is a natural outgrowth of the mutual frustrations experienced by these organizations as they have faced difficulties in maintaining adequate communication, trust, and cooperation between national and local units. The role of regional consultant is a difficult one. A consultant is in most instances physically and psychologically detached from the national office, but he can never be a full-fledged member of the local unit. Caught in some kind of interactional space between the two, the consultant faces demands from above and below. Often these pressures result in serious role conflict. Anyone who has worked with this kind of organizational structure is familiar with the typical complaints made about regional staff. The national office feels that the regional representative does not adequately understand and implement national programs. The temptation is for national staff to bypass the regional office and move directly into the field to exert influence on state and local units. The local units, from their perspective, complain that the regional staff either does not tell them what to do or it attempts to overdirect local activities, and thus is not as helpful as it should be. A regional consultant, far from being a helper, may be viewed as a snooper who sets himself up to judge the adequacy of local activities. Yet, despite all of these built-in problem potentials, regional office structures are in many instances a highly effective means for vertical integration.

A further means of vertical integration is provided by certain individuals within most communities of any size who tend to be oriented toward community life at the regional, state, or national level. These are the cosmopolitans mentioned earlier. They read national publications; they view local problems from the perspecive of more complex concerns at the national or even the international level; and they find opportunities to interact with their counterparts from other sections of the country. In addition to informal contacts, the cosmopolitan is likely to be found on regional or national committees and study commissions working on social problems, and with governmental authorities established to coordinate and administer programs. Like the regional staff person, the cosmopolitan faces the problem of a split and often conflicting identity. As his network of personal or professional associations outside the local community becomes both extensive and personally rewarding, he may find himself becoming alienated from local leaders within his community. It is difficult for such a citizen to adequately represent the local needs in regional or national circles. It is equally difficult for him to convey a national perspective to the local community. Yet it is terribly important in a complex, changing society that more and more people become able to fill this challenging role.

There is urgent need to strengthen and make more meaningful the link between local community life and the activities of those who must confront the complex regional, national, and international problems of our society. It must be emphasized that awareness of the difficulty is not enough; neither are good will and cooperative intent. What is required is competence—the ability of both professional and lay leaders to establish the conditions that will permit cooperative planning and action as well as the ability to resolve inevitable differences in perspective and point of view.

That community leadership skills can be augmented by training is borne out by the experiments in leadership training conducted by the National Training Laboratories of the National Education Association, (Mial and Mial, 1962). University centers for the behavioral sciences also have conducted leadership development programs that have led to improved problem solving and citizen action within and between communities. There are growing indications that the community-development field, for a long time focused mainly on work in emerging nations, has an important part to play in helping strengthen community life in

this country and to integrate local needs with national and regional resources (Franklin, 1966; Mial, 1958). There may, indeed, be a place for
a professional consultant on community life comparable to the position
of county agent in rural areas. In urban areas especially, such a community consultant, called by some the urban agent, may do much to
bring order out of chaos, strengthen the sense of community, and stimulate the development of both local and cosmopolitan leaders capable of
maintaining the integrity of the local community while linking effectively with both voluntary and governmental groups at regional and
national levels.

PLANNING AS AN INTEGRATIVE MECHANISM

A pervasive problem of social planning for housing, welfare, mental
health, or virtually any other area has been to relate the conceptual
schemes and dreams of the planners to the needs and motivations of the
individuals affected by their plans. Social planning cannot be successful
until this problem is resolved. Successful social planning is a necessity if
adequate horizontal and vertical integration of communities is to be
maintained. To understand these human obstacles in the way of successful planning, let us look first at some planning models.

The first model may be called rational planning. This approach
emphasizes the importance of assembling and organizing all available
data, which are then used by experts to arrive at overall plans as fully
developed and comprehensive as possible. Such planning is best carried
out by experts who are competent to make judgments in whatever sub-
stantive areas are involved. Laymen may be called on to sanction the
planning in the first place, to familiarize themselves with the plans once
they have been made, and to help influence the appropriate public officials who must in the end see to it that plans are implemented. For the
rational planner, the occasional irrationality which he finds in citizens,
pressure groups, legislative bodies, and others can be a major obstacle.
When faced with apparently irrational opposition, the planner attempts
to overcome it either by force of logic and argument or by engineering
consent through a public relations program.

An opposite approach to planning accepts from the outset the premise
that people much of the time will behave irrationally on the basis of
personal needs, values, and biases. This approach suggests that planning
at best can only be an accommodation to the diverse interests and
prejudices of those involved. The job of the expert then is to salvage as
much rationality as possible from the maelstrom of conflicting interests

and viewpoints. The frustrations can be enormous when, as one mental health administrator puts it, the orderly plans resulting from careful surveys stand in sharp contrast with the "disorderly possibles" that are the realities of the administrator's life (Schwartz, 1965).

A more realistic approach to planning is based on the acceptance of personal needs, human motivation, value differences and the like, as part of the social reality within which planning must proceed. It assumes that no plan made by experts, however capable, will be any more than an approximation of what in the end will prove to be both most practical and desirable (Demone, 1965). In this approach the initial planning involves a synthesis of the expertise of the planner and the knowledge of local needs, customs, and the like, which can only be provided by those who are to be affected by the plans themselves. One of the most important tasks of the planner is to find ways to enter into effective collaboration with local lay and professional groups. The planning process then becomes open to repeated inputs from these groups. Preliminary formulations by the planners are tested against their reactions and modified where necessary. By the time final plans are arrived at, they are more fully grounded in the realities of the local situation, and are therefore more likely to be put into operation.

Methods of group consultation are especially useful in bringing together workers, whether from the same or different agencies involved with the same client or sets of clients (Kevin, 1963; Rieman, 1963; Altrocchi et al., 1965). As Altrocchi and colleagues point out, group consultation has a double advantage over individual consultation in that it brings about a more complete and integrative understanding of a case and fosters improved interagency cooperation.

It is evident that professionals in the mental health field have moved rapidly during the past decade to the more realistic approach of planning with laymen. Citizens in catchment areas are being involved in many cases from the beginning, in advisory or policy boards, to help determine local needs, to link the professionals with area groups, and to interpret to residents the nature and limitations of staff resources available to them.

There remain those who hold stubbornly to the belief—common among health professionals over the years—that mental health planning should be left to the experts, however. As a resource consultant to a number of conferences on board-staff relationships in mental hygiene clinics prior to 1960, I became aware that professional distrust of the layman was strongly implanted. To many of the professionals citizen boards were an unnecessary nuisance that could only siphon off scare staff time and interfere with professional prerogatives.

In some cases a crisis will unfreeze attitudes or generate the motivation to involve the local resident in the affairs of the center.

The Los Angeles County mental health program, a large and well-established resource, moved rapidly in the direction of collaborative planning after the Watts disorders. Its director and other staff members were led by the violence to confront the possibility that their services were not equally available to all county residents. As the director later pointed out, although the clinics in the Watts area were always busy, there was growing doubt that they were being used by those "too fearful, too alienated, too hopeless" to seek help (Brickman, 1967, p. 649).

THE INTEGRATING ROLE OF THE MENTAL HEALTH WORKER

Mental health personnel have the potential to play an important integrative role in their communities. Being consultants to various groups, they are in an excellent position to spot breakdowns in communication and other barriers that vitiate effective intracommunity collaboration. Although *in* the community, they are not so much *of* it—that is, so embedded within the matrix of local biases—to be unable also to facilitate needed integration with state, regional, and national resources. Usually all that is needed is for the consultant to play a catalytic role. By asking questions such as, "Have you discussed this problem with (X)?" or, "Do you think (X) would have some ideas about this situation?" he may help the consultee move through barriers against contact caused by ignorance, narrowness of vision, or fear and bias. In some situations the mental health worker can be most helpful by bringing together individuals or groups whose collective wisdom may be needed if a particular problem is to be dealt with adequately. The job of the worker may be to convene the group and to help define the problem in such a way that the relevance of the several resources becomes apparent to all concerned. He may also need to stand ready to intervene as a group process resource in case conflicts arise or the climate of the discussion threatens to block frank and open exploration of the problem. It is important that the worker not enter such a meeting with his own solution to the problem. If he has a solution to suggest, he must be ready to modify or relinquish it in light of the group's deliberations.

As we have seen, integrative mechanisms, however adequate they may be in the day-to-day life of the community, may break down in the face of a crisis or emergency situation. When passions arise, there is pressure for action accompanied by dissatisfaction or distrust of the usual deliberative and problem solving procedures.

Vigilante justice is an example of such a breakdown. Pressures from citizens to "throw the book" at juvenile delinquents or to require loyalty oaths of teachers are other instances. Sometimes in a conflict situation the mental health worker himself may be pressured to take a stand on a vital moral issue such as civil rights, which he himself may believe has mental health implications. Although he may empathize with the sense of urgency experienced by any pressure group, the worker may need to indicate when he feels that proposed action solutions are not founded either on adequate diagnosis or on consideration of all available alternatives. Even if he chooses to emphasize the relevance for mental health of a proposal, he can still remain in a position to foster sober reflection and coordinated community action. Granted that sometimes it is possible to do so only after premature, ill-considered actions have been tried and found to be inadequate.

A highly imaginative and carefully documented instance of intervention for improved community integration has been carried out by Leighton and his colleagues (Beiser, 1965; A. Leighton, 1965). Using widely accepted group action techniques of community development, they brought about increased community integration (as measured by the same indices used in their original survey ten years before) and a concomitant reduction in the prevalence rate of impairing psychiatric disorders. Their experience underscores the importance of developing a basic minimum of community integration *as a precondition* for the later delivery of more sophisticated psychiatric resources (Beiser, 1965, p. 76).

The mental health worker is helped to be alert to potential interventions on the side of intracommunity coordination as well as vertical integration by becoming familiar with common potential cleavage points in organizational and community life (e.g., conflict between the generations often makes it difficult for adults and adolescents to consult with one another on problems of mutual concern). As suggested earlier, frictions are endemic between local, regional, and national representatives of the same organization. Also frequent in voluntary associations are difficulties surrounding problems of authority and control between staff and volunteer leadership. The list also includes the barriers to communication and understanding to be found between ethnic, racial, and religious groups, as well as inbuilt conflict in relations between labor and management. In fact, in any situation where there is a division of labor or responsibility, there are apt to arise misunderstandings and stereotypic responses based on difficulties in taking the role of the other.

When faced with a particular instance of breakdown in relations, the mental health worker may be in a position to help move the discussion to a more general consideration of the nature of the cleavage. In this way he may be able to help those involved lift the problem out of the level of personality differences or discussion of the inadequacies of the antagonists. It may then be possible to begin to delineate the more basic aspects of the problem and to determine how the cleavage can best be handled.

Methods of participative learning and problem solving developed by behavioral scientists involved in group dynamics or human relations training have proved extremely helpful as groups have sought to understand and do something about the kinds of cleavages in question (Bradford et al., 1964, Schein and Bennis, 1966). Contact alone, while sometimes helpful, is often not enough. Without adequate attention to the nature of the experience and how all concerned may learn from it, contact may even worsen the situation and make integration more difficult than before.

New roles within mental health and other programs are also being tried. While some are intended only to provide a badly needed source of manpower (e.g., the growing number of junior college programs for the training of mental health technicians) discussed by Hadley and True, 1968), others are seeking to enhance the utilization of mental health services by specific marginal groups. Subprofessional workers drawn from the same socioeconomic and ethnic groups as their clients are often more trusted by and better able to communicate with those in need of help than are more socially distant highly trained, middle-class professionals (Reiff and Riessman, 1966). Similarly, former mental patients are in an excellent position to help those returning from mental hospitals cope with the myriad problems of rehabilitation. The traditional team is rapidly being expanded to include a variegated phalanx of case aides, expeditors, indigenous nonprofessionals, and quasi-ombudsmen, all of whom have in common the one virtue of being able to bridge the gap between marginal man and the establishments seeking to help him.

Whatever methods are used, one of the most vital contributions to effective community problem solving that the mental health worker can make (and therefore one of the most important contributions to mental health) is to help strengthen the means whereby differences are resolved and cleavages are overcome both within the community and among it and the groups outside with which it must deal. For, it seems to me, we run the risk of substituting new roles and new program packages for more substantial and prolonged efforts to analyze and eliminate the forces which have led to and are sustaining cleavage, marginality, and disintegration. Indeed, the very act of creating new roles or new programs may enable existing professional groups and agencies to continue their work as before and thus to avoid the discomforts which would accompany efforts to modify their own procedures and perspectives. As

Gordon has suggested, the relatively rapid development of Head Start and high school dropout programs may be accounted for by the fact that they require little change in the school itself. Gordon (1965, p. 647) is being more realistic than cynical, I believe, when he says that it is often "easier to add extensions than to change the basic structure of institutions."

5

The Community as an Arena for Action

"The call of action has long been with me; not action derived from thought, but rather flowing from it in one continuous sequence. And when, rarely, there has been full harmony between the two, thought leading to action and finding its fulfillment in it, action leading back to thought and a fuller understanding—then I have sensed a certain fullness of life and a vivid intensity in that moment of existence."

JAWAHARLAL NEHRU, The Discovery of India (1946, p. 10).

CHAPTER SIXTEEN

The Development of Pressures for Action

The community so far has been discussed as a social system where inter-action occurs between people and values; where needs are met and a vast array of functions performed; where change occurs while integration is maintained; and where power is distributed, conflicts managed and decisions made. Within these complexities most people find some semblance of order and patterning to their existence. Implicit in all of the above has been the attempts by various individuals and groups to achieve their ends through purposive social action. The mental health movement is made up of such groups, and the mental health worker is caught up in a social action context which he needs to understand and be aware of as he goes about his activities. The mental health worker confronts the dynamic of community action most directly whenever he becomes a collaborator or action leader. At other times he may be treating, consulting with, seeking to educate and inform, or collaborating with others who themselves are part of a community action process.

The subject of community action has fascinated community sociologists for years. How do problem areas emerge for community consideration? What factors determine which of the many problems will capture people's attention and energies? Why are some groups more successful than others in translating their concerns into action? Applied to mental health concerns, such questions arise as the following: What are the most effective ways to bring problems to citizens' attention? What determines whether or not people will be convinced of the need for new or enlarged mental health services? How can the mental health staff best move from the point of its concern with a problem, such as a necessity for treatment facilities for juvenile offenders, to the point at which others also have become concerned and the needed facilities finally set up?

Such questions cannot be answered either simply or categorically. There are few sure prescriptions for community action. Nevertheless there are some caveats to be kept in mind; and there is a patterning to community action that, if perceived, can help the worker select more wisely from among alternative actions.

THE SEQUENCE OF ACTION

A sequence of community action must begin with a person who believes that a need or problem exists. Occasionally the response is to a new need or problem. In most instances, however, the problem has existed over a considerable period of time and has only just been "discovered" by the individual. Often the availability of new information leads to the recognition of a need and to the beginning of community action (e.g., many people rediscovered major and minor emotional disorders more or less simultaneously during and immediately after World War II in the United States). One reason seems to have been that new information about draft rejections and breakdown under combat stress dramatized the social implications of mental illness.

Awareness of need often becomes focused because new, more effective means of coping with a problem are discovered. Probably most of the impetus for the concentration on mental health as an area for community action after World War II arose from the successful large-scale application of psychiatric screening and treatment methods by the military, and later within the Veterans Administration. It is understandable that people do not mobilize for action on a social problem for which no solution is apparent. Conversely, it is more possible for a problem to be "discovered" if some way to begin working on it is available. It seems that good solutions find their own problems.

Perhaps it is even more apt to say that solutions sometimes become problems (i.e., the emergence of a problem for community action often occurs in terms of some way of dealing with it). The problem is defined in the context of the solution that is being proposed. In recent years, for example, most community action efforts concerned with the prevention of dental caries have emerged in terms of fluoridation of public water supplies as the ultimate solution. In mental health, too, the initial expression of social need usually occurs on the basis of some means for its solution.

Some years ago I worked with a small, newly developed group of citizens intent on establishing a mental health facility in their county. It quickly became apparent that the expression of need for each of the five people involved was almost exclusively in terms of a particular solution to a particular problem. For one the problem was the provision of treatment services for alcoholics; for another a court clinic for the treatment of juvenile delinquents; for a third a diagnostic and treatment service for children and their families, and so on. For each member of the group, the recognition of need and the concern about the problem were manifested in terms of the solution to be sought. Each individual had done considerable research into his solution and, in so doing, had become a kind of specialist on alcohol treatment programs, court clinics, child guidance facilities, etc. Moreover, having become committed to a problem definition based on a specific solution, each was quite resistant to efforts at broader exploration of mental health needs in general.

SOURCES OF ACTION PRESSURES

Initial recognition of a community need or problem often is accompanied by considerable pressure for reaching solutions. For every cause in the community there is at least one individual with a "bee in the bonnet." The urgency for action may be at the level of the individual, the group or organization, or the community as a whole. Of these, the urgency within the individual is readily understood by the mental health worker in motivational terms. It was not difficult to recognize the individual motivations of each member of the mental health group mentioned in the preceding. In fact the group members themselves were aware that their sense of urgency arose either from their own personal conflicts or problems faced by friends or relatives. Each of these people had a "bee in the bonnet." If not, they probably would not have come together in the first place. Nor would they have persevered through months of slow and frustrating efforts to reach agreements and to gain support from the community.

Entire groups and organizations can respond with similar urgency to their discovery of a need. Their commitment is total; the problem is preeminent over all others; the solution is known; it is pursued with insistence and single-mindedness that sometimes cannot fathom why other groups do not become equally committed. Examples of such organizational urgency can be found in the mental health movement, certain political organizations, and a wide variety of other groups committed to causes of various sorts. Usually they, too, have hit on solutions to be sought (e.g., fluoridation, prohibition, impeachment of a Supreme Court Judge) which they feel will take care of the problem that concerns them. The urgency stems in part from the conviction that the problem is critical, in part from the fact that the solution has been found.

Urgency that is community-wide occurs less often. It involves concern on the part of many or most of the citizens and usually reflects a sense of crisis, an actual or imagined threat to the community's well-being. The loss of a major industry, destruction of large neighborhood areas because of highway construction, and the rapid influx of strange newcomers, are examples of situations which have induced community-wide crises. Here again, communities typically respond with a statement of the problem founded on specific ways of solving it. In fact, such a sense of community-wide urgency that presses for one or more specific solutions is itself symptomatic of a community crisis.

> The citizens of a suburban community were profoundly upset by a series of suicides and fatal automobile accidents involving teenagers that occurred in the space of just a few months. Strong pressures developed to raise the legal state minimum driving age. Intense efforts to influence the state authorities persisted for several months despite motor vehicle registry data which indicated that older teenagers and young adults were those groups most often involved in fatal accidents. Attempts by a mental health team to involve those most concerned in a consideration of the underlying causes of adolescent distress or of measures to provide more community supports for teenagers were rejected. Only after the crisis had spontaneously eased was it possible to approach some of the community's problems with respect to its adolescents in a more comprehensive, systematic fashion.

Community action, then, arises from the commitment both to a problem and its probable solution. Yet, such single-minded commitment to action too often results in inadequate assessment of the problem, neglect of alternative solutions, and even the alienation of potential supporters.

THE IMPORTANCE OF TIMING

Though conviction and commitment are necessary for successful action, like love in child-rearing, they are not enough. A factor analytic study of seventeen successful and unsuccessful cases of community development provides some leads as to possible reasons for their success or failure (Janes, 1961). Predictive of success was a complex of characteristics including (a) degree of involvement of local people in the project, and (b) careful professional planning and preparation. Factors associated with failure were not nearly as clear-cut, though the presence of factionalism before a project was initiated, inability to develop new community leadership during the course of a project, and an impersonal and inflexible presentation of project aims seemed to be associated with lack of success in some efforts.

Also needed are accurate timing and an awareness that certain steps are needed in order to move successfully from the "bee in the bonnet" phase to the ultimate achievement of solutions acceptable to a community. Specialists in community action and theory have described various models for understanding and relating to community action. All have recognized that, given the complexity of community dynamics, any such model oversimplifies and only approximates real life. By providing an abstract guide to analysis of real situations, it can help those who use it to make wiser decisions about their own behavior. As Mial (1961, p. 86) puts it:

"At least it is possible to indicate the need for timing, for awareness of process, for patience in *planning* before rushing into action. It (the action model) may help to focus on points of frequent breakdown. It may be possible to increase, to some extent, the predictability of results. And it may help to encourage comparative discussion of different approaches. Above all, it may help to encourage men of action to analyze what they are doing and to keep records of efforts and results."

CHAPTER SEVENTEEN

Steps in Community Action

AN IDEALIZED MODEL

The famous sociologist Eduard Lindemann is generally credited with the first systematic attempt to develop a model for community action from the study of actual cases. Lindemann's "steps in community action" (E. C. Lindemann, 1921) are essentially descriptive. They do not go as far as more recent efforts, which are presented later, to analyze distinctive phases and underlying processes. It is apparent that Lindemann, like some of those who have followed him in the analysis of community action, also tended to view the sequence as an idealized model for how action should proceed rather than simply as an empirical description. Briefly stated, his ten steps were:

1. Expression of need;
2. Spreading the awareness of need within some grouping;
3. Projection of consciousness of need upon community leadership;
4. Impulse to meet need quickly;
5. Presentation of solutions;
6. Conflict of solutions;
7. Investigation of solutions with expert assistance;
8. Open discussion;
9. Emergence of a practicable solution;
10. Compromise on basis of tentative progress.

ACTION STEPS AND THE STANCE OF THE MENTAL HEALTH AGENCY

Lindemann's analysis can be used to point up certain basic aspects of community action. The first of these is the movement from an original recognition of a problem to spreading the awareness within a more or less restricted group or organization. This would appear to be one of the most critical early transition points in nascent community action. At this point, those initially concerned are seeking validation for their concern through the interest, support, and perhaps involvement of those with whom they feel most comfortable and whose judgment they are apt to respect. If from somewhere within this immediate circle of relatives, friends, people of like mind, or friendly experts there is not some encouragement, the sequence probably will not continue.

Only rarely are mental health specialists consulted at the initial phase. Consultation at this point, when it does occur, however, might well be focused on what has been done to explore others' interests. It is important, for example, to determine whether the individual's immediate circle of acquaintances has been consulted and, if so, whether they have supported his concern. It seems unlikely that professional interest and support from the mental health agency alone would be sufficient encouragement without some convergence of concern among fellow citizens.

Mental health specialists are more apt to be consulted after convergence has occurred and a group has formed to work on a problem. Expert help at such a time may be helpful, especially if the consultees are interested in gathering further data about the nature and extent of the problem. Very often, however, the consultees' motivations are uncertain or unrealistic and clarification of the help being sought is needed. Often a group at this phase is seeking allies, not professional consultation. It may believe that the mental health facility has much influence in the community and should take the lead in bringing about the desired result. It might be seeking to enlist expert authority to line up on its side against anticipated opposition. The power of a mental health agency, as we have seen, is rarely sufficient to overcome the barriers to community action. Therefore it is important to clarify what action, if any, the agency can undertake and what kind of help is being offered.

As action moves from steps three to five, the sense of urgency frequently takes over. Groups may wish to bypass all further attempts to diagnose and assess alternatives. If the mental agency does not become an ally or is not powerful enough to effect action, the group may turn to others, such as the clergy, political leadership, prestige figures, or mass media in an effort to short circuit action and find a speedy means of meeting the need. Such efforts usually fail. They are founded on an inadequate development of a base of community understanding and support among those groups and institutions most directly related to the problem at hand. Community action efforts are sometimes abandoned at just this point. The protagonists retire from the field, frustrated, angry, and discouraged; often they project responsibility for defeat on those in positions of power and influence who, in the eyes of the initiators, have refused to place their powers at the group's disposal. To forestall unnecessary defeat, the mental health team may be able to keep alive the possibility of action by helping the group develop the more realistic perspective that would enable it to take the action needed to continue its efforts.

Three aspects of community action are not covered in Lindemann's analysis. These are (a) securing the approval and support needed to make the action and the group supporting it a legitimate part of the community (a process called by different authors sanction, sponsorship, or legitimation), (b) developing an appropriate organizational base for action, and (c) evaluating the action sequence by a more or less continuous process in order to modify goals and approaches as needed.

Mental health agencies sometimes are asked to endorse a community effort which, in its protagonists' eyes, is relevant to mental health. The mental health agency, however, is a professionally oriented institution which rarely is part of the central decision making circles of a community. Its endorsement alone infrequently constitutes an acceptable sanction for a proposed activity or the group proposing it. If the staff wishes to support a proposal, however, it may help the action group to identify and involve those institutions and key individuals whose combined approval may be needed before the next step can be taken.

If a proposal has mental health implications, the mental health facility may be asked to implement it rather than simply to provide legitimation. In most cases, however, it is best to determine the ultimate organizational base only after developing the needed sanction. Having developed it, the question of organizational base can be faced more realistically. Perhaps the other groups involved will accept the mental health facility as the proper agency. On the other hand, it may be necessary to develop a shared responsibility by locating resources within two or more organizations. In some cases, an entirely new organization must be developed, supported by but separate from those whose sponsorship has made it possible.

Such a decision is best made by joint deliberations on the part of all those involved. Obviously, no one should be allowed to thrust an unwanted responsibility on the professional staff of a mental health center; neither should others be able to keep the mental health team from undertaking responsibilities it deems both desirable and within its professional purview. The community action model does suggest, nonetheless, that unilateral action by the mental health team either to accept or reject a new responsibility usually will run unnecessarily high risks; these risks may in the end jeopardize community understanding and support of a program.

The desirability of building evaluation into any community action sequence is apparent to most scientifically trained mental health specialists. Yet in practice even the most rudimentary efforts at evaluation are sometimes neglected by community mental health teams. Why is this so? Perhaps it is because the community is unfamiliar territory; the phenomena are complex, and it is not possible with any certainty to determine what criteria for success should be used, which of the many dimensions are most important for study, and how best to study them. Another formidable obstacle can be the rigorous scientific standards for inquiry brought by team members themselves. Community action situations rarely can be studied in ways that would satisfy most researchers. Few, if any, objective measures are possible in such fluid circumstances, and usually it is not feasible to undertake comparative or controlled observations of several settings.

Handled properly, evaluation of community action can serve as a useful aid to those involved. Ideally, data collection and feedback should be attempted at every step along the way. The information sought should be of the kind that will facilitate understanding of the goals being sought, the extent to which those involved believe that progress has been made toward their goals, and their perceptions of problems still to be faced, steps to be taken, and the like. This kind of evaluation research is incorporated within the action system itself; the data, which are made available to all concerned, are part of the mechanism which determines the appropriate steps to be taken.

A WORKING MODEL FOR COMMUNITY ACTION

The following model for community action is taken from Sower's work in programs involving social scientists in community related projects (Sower, 1957). It is chosen in preference to others for three reasons: first, it attempts to conceptualize the interplay between citizens and consultants and therefore seems especially useful to the mental health worker; second, it recognizes that the nature and flow of action is a function of community attitudes and characteristics as well as the strategy and orientation of the action group; third, it formulates broad phases and so permits considerable variation in specifics from one situation to another. The seven phases in the model are: (a) convergence of interest, (b) initiation of action, (c) legitimation and sponsorship, (d) development of an overall plan, (e) development of a suitable organization for action, (f) implementation, and (g) evaluation (viewed, as indicated earlier, as an integral part of the action system throughout its course). It was suggested earlier that community action groups often attempt to shortcut the process by eliminating one or more phases or overlooking essential steps to be taken within any action phase. Stated in summary fashion, the following are some of the more common "mistakes" which can lead to blocked action and unnecessary failure to attain objectives:

WITHIN THE CONVERGENCE OF INTEREST PHASE

1. Those involved become too quickly discouraged by initial lack of response on the part of those with whom interest is tested;

2. They do not recognize interest when it does exist, sometimes because they are not ready to modify their objectives or purposes in order to make it possible to converge with the motivations and goals of others;

3. They do not spread the net widely enough, thus overlooking groups that are vitally concerned with the problem in question;

4. They do not look into the history of the problem within the community to determine the extent to which efforts to deal with it have been tried in the past and with what consequences;

5. They do not make appropriate use of available consultative help, often out of ignorance that such help exists either within the local community, at neighboring universities, or from the state and national agencies.

WITHIN THE INITIATION OF ACTION PHASE

1. Those involved fail to recognize sources of potential assistance or include them in the initial planning;

2. They do not recognize sources of potential opposition and take them into account;

3. They create unnecessary static by not including in the planning process groups already involved in related activities;

4. They are unwilling to turn over primary responsibility for the succeeding action steps to an existing organization better suited to the purpose, with the result that the problem becomes caught up in an intergroup or interagency conflict.

WITHIN THE LEGITIMATION AND SPONSORSHIP PHASE

1. Those involved do not indicate that they are concerned with whether their needs and purposes deserve high priority within existing community goals and resources;

2. They do not make an adequate assessment of the ways in which decisions are made in their community, do not identify appropriate decision makers, and do not develop effective contacts with them;

3. They insist that potential sponsors accept a specific action plan or program, rather than beginning by soliciting interest in the problem area itself;

4. They incorrectly decide they have sufficient power to override opposition from established community decision makers, and so proceed without needed legitimation;

5. They overlook sources of power that can help them neutralize opposition and secure implicit sanction from those who might otherwise be openly opposed.

WITHIN THE PHASE OF DEVELOPMENT OF AN OVERALL PLAN

1. Those involved do not make it possible for procedures for planning to be carefully thought through and decided on by all concerned;

2. They do not deal with tensions that develop between the original initiators and the enlarged group as issues arise about who will exert most influence;

3. They develop a plan that fails to take into account procedures that would secure information about the problem needed to identify various possible action steps, and to determine community attitudes toward the problem and its solution;

4. They fail to take into account the needs and attitudes of those most likely to be directly affected by possible action steps as well as others whose interests also are likely to be involved;

5. They become unwilling to entertain possible redefinition of their goals or procedures because pressures for arriving at a decision are so intense;

6. They allow the interest of participants to diminish as fewer and fewer people take ever greater responsibility for the group's work;

7. They fail to take into account possible sources of support and opposition;

8. They devote insufficient time and effort to handling suspicions and other tensions within the group or between themselves and outsiders.

1. Those involved do not identify or take into account the concerns and vested interests of existing organizations;

2. They do not seek to determine all possible existing organizations to be considered in making a selection;

3. They develop such pride of ownership in the plan that it becomes impossible for them to consider handing over their proposal for implementation by others;

4. They let their desire for results render them unrealistically optimistic or pessimistic about their own resources to do the job (or about others' resources to take it over);

5. They develop premature discouragement because of difficulties in securing an action base within an existing organization, with the result that the group fails to consider the possibility of developing a new organization to confront data that are contrary to their preconceptions and convictions;

6. They treat the results of evaluation only as indicators of relative success or failure, rather than as information from which they can learn to improve their efforts;

7. They maintain inadequate records of the activities at every step along the way, with the result that it is not possible to relate outcomes to the action processes themselves.

LIMITATIONS OF THE ACTION MODEL

Like most sets of guidelines, the action model appears deceptively simplistic. It pulls together into a few temporal phases all the complexities, passions, and frustrations of a process that may involve the efforts of scores of people over the course of many months or years. It is, after all, primarily a statement in community terms of a basic orientation to problem solving. How can it do justice to, or serve as a guide for, intricacies of community involvement? Just because of its categorical simplicity, it has the merit of enabling the mental health worker to organize rapidly shifting and complex interactions into a meaningful pattern. Used thoughtfully and creatively, it can focus the interventions of the mental health team selectively on the most pertinent concern facing those with whom it consults.

As suggested earlier, it can help the mental health center determine whether and in what manner to enter into an action effort: either as (a) the original concerned group, (b) among the converging band of initiators, (c) part of the later larger circle of those planning for action, (d) included in the legitimating body that puts the seal of approval on the emerging action program, (e) as implementers of part or all of a final action plan, or (f) as contributors to the evaluation process. Like other such contrivances, the action model will not be very helpful if used rigidly or in a mechanical way. It is certainly true that real-life community-action sequences are rarely as clear-cut as the model implies. Certain phases may extend over months or even years; others are over in only a few days; still others may take place outside the purview of the mental health worker altogether. In some cases the sequence of steps may be altered.

The model takes into account only a single action sequence, whereas there are innumerable intersecting action sequences occurring at any one time in a given community. Interests between action groups converge and diverge; alliances are formed or competition develops. Efforts and energies shift from one objective to another. Action sequences collide and cancel one another out or reinforce one another. An adequate model for describing the interplay of action efforts in the community has yet to be developed. Until it is available, it is possible to use what we have as a simplified approximation of the vastly more complex reality with which the mental health team must deal in any community action.

CHAPTER EIGHTEEN

Orientation of the Mental Health Agency to the Community

"Our task is *not* to copy Athens but to work toward a city in our technological age which puts the education of free, thinking, responsible, participating, aesthetically sensitive, justly critical citizens as the ultimate measure of its success or failure, its maturity or immaturity."

KENNETH BENNE, *Criteria of a Mature Community.*

An elderly juvenile court judge a few years ago took time out to participate in an intensive one-week human relations training experience. Asked whether he had learned anything from the experience, the judge commented, "After being on the bench so many years, I had about forgotten that I have an effect on people. You know, I'm going to have to go home and look into that!" [12]

In the mental health field we have known for a long time that we have had an effect on people. It remains now for us to determine what kind of effect it is both possible and desirable to have as mental health resources become increasingly comprehensive and community-related.

This volume has sought to impress the reader with the richness and importance of community life to the individual and to the mental health field. It has suggested in many different ways that the mental health agency and its professional staff have the potential for affecting not only individuals within the community, but also the very quality of community life itself. In fact, to the extent that the agency seeks to promote well-being and reduce the incidence of emotional disorders, it must devote careful attention to influencing community patterns. What is it that this book suggests might be "looked into" if mental health

[12] Dr. Charles Seashore, NTL Institute for Applied Behavioral Science: personal communication.

agencies are to realize their potential as influencers of environmental change?

I proposed at the outset that it is desirable to cultivate an appreciation of the range and richness of community institutions and processes. The sense of community possessed by many mental health workers is limited by the restricted scope of contacts with community groups during the typical course of training and traditional work experience. Needed most of all is a lively sense of curiosity coupled with a willingness to explore the many different groups and institutions making up any community. Rather than limiting our excursions to contacts with the more obvious community allies such as clergymen, physicians, social workers, public health nurses, and educators, for example, we should be willing to venture farther afield. This means we can explore possible points of interest convergence with such other groups as county agents, law enforcement officials, adult educators, librarians, personnel people in business and industry, labor officials, community planners, chamber of commerce executives, and newspaper people. The list could be extended further to include less obvious caretakers of particular groups, as, for example, the bartender and his tavern, if we are concerned for the well-being of homeless men (Dumont, 1967). The main point, however, is to cultivate a sense of community that is alert to the virtually endless variety of ways in which mental health concerns are dealt with and in which the mental health facility can link with, influence, and learn from the approaches of others.

THE TRANSITIONAL NATURE OF CURRENT MENTAL HEALTH WORK

The mental health worker has the problem of balancing a responsible desire to do what he knows best by making use of his specialized, unique competences, against a willingness to risk some possible role diffusion through a partial redefinition of what he can and must do to further the cause of mental health. The trained psychotherapist cannot confine himself exclusively to treatment without abandoning the commitment to have a meaningful impact on community life (unless, of course, he somehow restricts his practice to political leaders and other key influentials). On the other hand, the mental health worker's ticket of admission to the community in the first place usually has been his presumed ability to work intimately and directly with troubled and troublesome individuals. The field has been growing through what, in my opinion, is a kind of transition phase in which, with some few outstanding exceptions, the first tentative ventures into the community have been made from a largely clinical basis. Without surrendering much of the medico-clinical orientation, mental health workers have adopted the quasi-clinical tool of mental health consultation. Instead of a psychotherapist-patient relationship, they have developed a range of consultant-consultee relationships which, with some minor modifications of stance and perspective, have enabled the clinician to maintain pretty much his accustomed specialist orientation to those seeking his help.

I label this phase a transitional one because the implication of this volume's analysis of community processes calls for a major redefinition of the mental health agency, its scope and functions. Intimations of this redefinition, interestingly enough, are more often found in isolated examples of mental health programs within other settings, such as school systems and antipoverty programs, than within current institutional trends of mental health itself. The present development of comprehensive mental health centers in fact represents a peculiarly regressive trend to expand and, admittedly, improve direct treatment services at a time when many non-mental health groups are caught up in the exciting possibilities for more vital community-oriented efforts. Calling them community centers does not disguise the fact that in their prescribed functions they are rarely, if at all, committed to any important efforts at environmental modification and community change. The very guidelines for establishing community mental health centers under present federal legislation (P.L. 88–164) are insular and lacking in the flexibility required if the unique problems of individual communities are to be met (Hargrove, 1967).

Nonetheless, there is reason for optimism. As Ozarin (1966) points out, the history of public health facilities (as well as the demonstration Mental Health Study Center conducted by the National Institute of Mental Health in Prince George's County) shows that the existence of the public program stimulates the creation of other more specialized resources to care for certain disorders, and also attracts increased numbers of private practitioners able to take over some of the treatment burden. The public health facility then becomes freed to turn its attention toward community service functions and preventive activities. Thus it may well be that the current regression to a treatment and case-centered mode, by bringing mental illness back into the locality, is really in the service of the community ego. If so, we are truly in transition toward a comprehensive population-centered and preventively oriented mental health effort.

THE CHANGE AGENT FUNCTION

Ultimately, the overall goal of a community-oriented mental health center becomes that of community improvement. The major efforts and energies of the mental health team then become devoted to gaining a better understanding of basic community processes and to developing the means for making them more conducive to the emotional well-being of individuals.

Viewed from this perspective, the mental health worker becomes a conscious and deliberate agent of change who seeks to intervene at strategic points within subsystems of the community. He is guided in these efforts both by his appreciation of the unique quality and community-relatedness of the institution in question and by his vision of what the institution's potentialities are for the job of helping individuals achieve more effective skills of living. With this perspective it is not enough, for example (though it is certainly necessary), for the mental health worker to consult with school officials about the classroom management of a particular emotionally disturbed pupil. It is important that he or one of his colleagues in mental health also be concerned with far more basic mental health questions pertaining to the public schools. For example, what are the reasons why the ratio of boys to girls referred for emotional problems, reading disorders, classroom management problems and the like ranges from 2:1 to 4:1 in schools throughout the country? Or, what are the factors contributing to the endemic tensions existing between public school personnel and the public they serve, and what can be done to establish improved school-community relations?

The mental health worker draws as change agent from the growing body of knowledge and theory that has arisen from studies in small group and organizational change, alluded to at several points in this book, as well as the descriptions of the innovative process derived from work in such disparate areas as agriculture and medicine. Although he bases his interventions on social action techniques, however, he cannot afford to neglect the more traditional clinical and consultative models.

Some of the most innovative examples of the fusion of social action and traditional methodologies are to be found among new mental health programs in urban disadvantaged areas (e.g., Peck et al., 1966). In such areas of high need for immediate help, it is unrealistic and ineffective to work toward basic institutional changes without simultaneously providing markedly stepped up therapeutic and rehabilitative case-by-case services (Kahn, 1967).

A COMMUNITY–DEVELOPMENT ORIENTATION

Having accepted community improvement as his ultimate objective, the mental health worker also draws some part of his sustenance and role identity from the community-development field. He seeks to reduce the cleavages and distrust that Leighton, among others, found so clearly correlated with indices of social and emotional pathology. He finds ways to serve as an effective bridge between disparate and sometimes conflicting segments of the community, and as a link between the locally oriented concerns of residents and the regional, state, and national organizations with which the local community is linked for better or worse.

Perhaps most important, the mental health worker becomes a developer of human resources in the broadest possible sense. In so doing he takes on some of the responsibilities of the educator, allying himself whenever possible with the many adult educators of the community. He also tries in everything he does to identify, support, and cultivate the initiative and talents of potential community leadership. Training of volunteers and professionals for civic leadership is an essential part of any community action process. Efforts within mental health contexts to foster increased civic competence, unfortunately, have been virtually nonexistent. Mental health agencies have tended to limit their educational programs to increasing the screening, case-finding, referral, and counseling skills of professional groups. In Wellesley the approach was extended somewhat to involve a group of volunteers in a continuing effort to identify community concerns and communicate them to the board and staff of the agency and, conversely, to carry out both formal and informal efforts to interpret mental health needs and the work of the agency to key community groups.

In 1961, the Urban League of Washington, D.C. carried out an intensive leadership training laboratory for participants from forty-nine church, political, civil rights, business, labor, and neighborhood improvement organizations. Planned with the National Training Laboratories, this program sought to increase the ability of participants to work on specific problems across racial, religious, and economic barriers. Material on community theory and the particular characteristics of Washington was integrated with a focus on actual problems that needed to be considered at multiple levels, ranging from the encounters of individuals with each other at the workshop itself to the unique political realities of the city (Bellamy, 1962). Following the one-week workshops, participants continued to work together on three community improvement projects. Though not a mental health project, the workshop had self-development as one of its objectives, and included a psychiatrist, a professor of community organization, and an Urban League trainer on its staff, as well as National Training Laboratories' personnel.

Since 1961, other community groups have been involved in similar programs designed to increase collaboration across usual community barriers in a number of
cities, including Boston, New York City, Cincinnati, Kansas City, Chicago, Atlanta,
and Salt Lake City. Annual two-week summer residential workshops on community
leadership are offered under NTL auspices or with NTL cooperation in Atlanta;
Cedar City, Utah; Bethel, Maine; and Kansas City, Missouri. Laboratory methods
of training are rapidly being adapted to the special problems and dynamics of
community interaction. They offer excellent training grounds for mental health
teams themselves as well as the means whereby linkages can be forged between
mental health and other community groups.

As indicated in the chapter on integration, there is a wealth of
community development experiences in this country and overseas, dat-
ing back to the 1920's, from which to draw. In the mental health field
there is the example of Leighton's work in Nova Scotia, described earlier. However, with this major exception and a few as yet less extensive,
but no less exciting, efforts in some urban areas, the mental health
movement has left the community development vein largely unmined.
Partly in reaction to this neglect but also out of an overriding conviction concerning its value, this book has tended throughout to formulate
the discussion of issues and approaches in the context of community
development. No doubt the mental health programs throughout the
country will need to find those approaches to community development
which are most congenial and appropriate to the specific goals of mental
health. But it seems inescapable that we must concentrate a major portion of our energies on the rehabilitation of community life rather than
continue to squander them only on the more conservative intervention
in the lives of individual patients or even single institutions.

A recent unpublished prospectus for the Sound View Throgs Neck Community
Mental Health Center in New York prepared by Gilbert Levin (1967) envisions a
three-part consultation and education service whereby the full resources of the
center and other agencies can be brought to bear on potential trouble spots (e.g., a
school where racial tensions are brewing); consultations to caretakers can be provided; and various educational, human relations training, and other growth-
producing techniques for fostering creative expression can be used "to provide
growth and learning experiences for those individuals in the community who are
most capable of profiting from them and most likely to be able to use them in
affecting life in the community" (pp. 2–3).

THE ACTION RESEARCH ROLE

Part of the mental health agency's strength to the community is its informed capacity to perform an active research role. Behavioral scientists
on the mental health team have been trained to ask the right questions,

or at least to ask questions in the right way (i.e., the way which enables data to be gathered that may help to suggest answers). The mental health agency must ask its own questions of the community laboratory —questions concerning variations in the distribution of forms of emotional disorder and factors associated with them; ways in which mental health concerns are dealt with in the community; and even more basic, how people become deviant or marginal in the first place. But the agency also must be responsive to the community's concerns, helping to formulate these concerns in the most productive ways, and assisting in the collection and interpretation of data bearing on them.

The skills involved here are not only the usual ones having to do with research design and implementation. There are also the important considerations having to do with enlistment of citizen sanction and support for searching inquiry in the community laboratory, as well as the unique possibilities inherent in the task of feeding back research data in ways which community groups will find most useful when policies are being shaped and decisions made.

To the extent that he remains aware of the implications of his new role and of the intricacies of the environment in which he plays this role, the mental health worker today has an enormous opportunity to contribute to a better understanding of the community as an environment which influences the emotional well-being of those environed by it. Awareness is an essential quality in this effort; it is the readiness to attend to the many subtleties of community interaction and to search for possible patternings of events that may lead to new insights about the relationship between man and his environment.

Much depends, of course, on the readiness of mental health leaders, public officials, and citizens to sanction and finance well-designed inquiries, including extensive epidemiologic studies as well as field surveys, careful natural history observations, and continuous program evaluations. Yet there is also much to be said for the ordered observations of an interested mental health worker who, embedded in some segments of community life such as the schools, the courts, the poverty milieu, or the circle of government, observes and records the on-going events with an informed attention to the dynamics and implications of what he experiences.

To be useful, such observations must be carefully and painstakingly carried out, much as the early naturalists recorded their observations in the field. One difference is that the mental health worker is also a participant in the events he is studying; he has the unique opportunity to record and learn from his own reactions to the interactions in which he is involved. Having calibrated himself in his community role as carefully as the psychotherapist does in his setting, the mental health worker can begin to develop a rich and subtle appreciation for the unique roles and functions within the community of those with whom he works. As he formulates questions which he believes are important, he is in an excellent position to enlist the collaboration of those with whom he consults in seeking out the data he needs both from their own experiences and from the reactions of others.

RESPECT FOR COMMUNITY INTEGRITY

Not only do such new functions require modification of old skills and the development of new ones having to do with communication, change agentry, and group procedures, they also must necessarily be founded on a deep and thoroughgoing concern for and understanding of the integrity of the community (Rosenblum and Ottenstein, 1965). Without a respect for community processes, the mental health field's participation in community intervention and change runs the risk of being disruptive to the community's integration and problem solving efforts. Mental health workers are familiar enough with the necessity for psychotherapists to empathize with the values and concerns of the patients they are seeking to help. Nonpatients (be they professional colleagues, consultees from other disciplines, or nonprofessional citizen leaders) are equally responsive to the worker who is genuinely interested in their aims and aspirations for their community.

Respect for community integrity goes beyond the needed understanding of the roles, functions, programs, goals, and values within each of the key agencies and institutions of the community. It also embraces a concern for the quality of the basic processes which are fundamental to the community's welfare—by which I mean such things as the manner in which policy is shaped and decisions made, interactions between different groups are facilitated, communication of information and values is fostered, and leadership encouraged to develop and deal with the myriad problems of community life. By paying attention to the processes of community life, the mental health agency is in a favorable position to call the attention of others to the possible consequences of the processes that are being used in any given instance. For the most part, the agency can remain sufficiently neutral in instances of community action so that it can help the various protagonists gauge the effects of their behavior and possibly even develop strategies that in the long run will be more rather than less conducive to community integration.

Respect for community integrity must include a predilection to take into account the readiness of a community to move in one or another direction. Mental health needs may be met in a deprived community more appropriately by the establishment of child-welfare services than by a specialized mental health center. In a well-endowed community the most important thrust may be made via consultation to and coordination of the several agencies already in existence (Robinson, 1963). It is essential that different patterns of mental health programming be available so that such efforts complement rather than disrupt specific and widely varying social, economic, and help-giving characteristics of communities throughout the country.

Robinson cites the case of a small county of 35,000 people which was being urged to establish a mental health unit within its health department, assigning public health nurses to follow up discharged mental patients from the state hospital. The health department was beset by a serious rabies epidemic. The community was without adequate precommitment, public welfare, probation, or other basic resources. The psychiatric ward of the community was unused, due to the staff's fear of mental patients. Robinson comments, "I wondered whether a psychiatric clinic was the single answer" (1963, p. 613). The question might be more aptly put, "Was it any answer to local needs at all?"

In its own actions, too, the mental health agency has the opportunity to develop tactics and strategies which emphasize a concern for processes and the climate of community action, perhaps even giving them more significance than the specific goals for which the agency is working. The widest possible involvement of citizens in the development of agency policies and the establishment of mental health priorities is an important part of the agency's contribution to the well-being of the community. It not only ensures more relevant and more successful programs, it also helps create more informed and committed leadership able to bring new insights and skills to a wide range of community activities.

PROFESSIONAL–LAYMAN RELATIONSHIPS

In all such activities with citizens, the mental health agency is not immune from the problems of professional-lay relationships that are apparently so endemic in our society. The history of health movements is replete with instances of suspicions and conflicts between health leaders and the citizens who have sought to work with them. That such problems are by no means restricted to matters of health is demonstrated by the following account of difficulties experienced by Tyrone Guthrie, the famous theatrical figure, with the Board of the Scottish National Theatre Society in the 1920's. Guthrie (1959, p. 50) writes: "But there, again, the old weakness became apparent—a weakness, incidentally, which is surely endemic in lay committees directing the policy of enterprises in which they take a benign interest, but about which they have almost no technical knowledge—they knew, neither severally nor collectively, neither in precise nor even in general terms, what they really did want." It is one thing to create a citizen policy making or advisory body; it is another to deal patiently and openly with the problems of authority, control, and distrust that are virtually inevitable in any sustained relationship between professional staff and citizen group. And yet, it is absolutely essential, to the community and to the agency itself, that such problems be resolved.

I recall one confrontation between a psychotherapist and board member who was asking for case examples that might help him understand the objectives and procedures of crisis intervention. When the therapist refused to provide case material, even fictional or highly disguised instances, out of concern for patient confidentiality, the board member responded, "Doctor, if you have a board for this mental health center which you staff people trust, the agency will have a long and productive existence. If you have a board you don't trust, you may last a few years. But if you didn't have a board, I'd give you no more than six months."

In the resolution of the dilemmas posed by the preceding confrontation much was learned on both sides, and the agency emerged with an even stronger and more dedicated staff-board alliance than it had enjoyed for many years.

The approach to staff and citizen collaboration can be conceived as an effort to effect an optimal integration of the rational-technical and social-process dimensions alluded to in an earlier chapter. The staff can provide the most well thought through and scientifically based point of view to the matter in hand; the citizen group, however, is in the best position to provide insights into how people may be perceiving the problem and how they may react to a proposed agency approach to it. Solutions based on the rational-technical expertise of staff or on the social-process insights of the board alone are apt to be faulted in some significant way. It is up to the staff members to be aware of the need for such an integration to occur and to help work toward it.

The integrative stance of the mental health agency has a number of possible ramifications. Among other things, it means that the agency seeks whenever possible to be responsive to the diversity of the community, upholding the possibility that a community can be more truly integrative if it permits pluralism of attitudes, values, and goals. As already suggested, it means the agency is in an excellent position to engage, with those involved in community problem solving or conflict resolution, in attempts to define issues and concerns in new and hopefully more productive ways, and to discover new solutions. Closely related to this, it means there is an emphasis on helping individuals and groups see the possibility of trying out new methods and approaches that had not been thought of and were not part of the community's or their traditional problem solving patterns.

Basically, therefore, it means a qualitatively very different contract between the mental health team and community groups from those usually negotiated between professionals and clients, in which the transaction is one of enhancing growth and change for both parties, rather than dependency and relative incompetence for a target group as it attempts to conform to the superior group's standards (Pratt and Tooley, 1966).

THE MENTAL HEALTH AGENCY AS AN INNOVATIVE RESOURCE

The agency also provides an innovative and experimental resource, willing itself to try out and evaluate new programs or to stimulate other groups to do so. Related, as mental health agencies usually are, to a number of associations and organizations outside the locality, their staffs can also devote some time and attention to looking toward the future in order to anticipate predicaments that the community may be facing because of probable changes that will be taking place.

In all of these activities and stances (i.e., the change agent, community development, action research, integrative and linking, and future-scanning) the staff of a mental health facility may be helped to maintain perspective and determine priorities by keeping in mind the essential nature of the community itself. It is very likely, as was pointed out in the opening section of this volume, to be the most essential context in which mankind functions. It is the community that reflects man-in-environment, the environment in which man interacts with other men in the quest for the significance that makes life worthwhile; and the environment that, throughout the individual's life cycle, determines the extent to which his needs are met and his problems resolved. The arrival of the mental health agency on the scene cannot help but affect this man-in-environment matrix; whether for better or worse depends on many things, not the least of which is the mental health worker's readiness to examine himself and question his ultimate role in relation to the complexities and challenges of the community itself.

I have sought in several ways to make the point that although the mental health team usually cannot abdicate the responsibility to provide specialized diagnostic, treatment, and rehabilitation services, it can and must find ways to foster those processes that are the very qualities of community excellence. These qualities are reflected in the behavior and characteristics of the citizens that are nurtured by the community. The citizens of the community to which the mental health movement can be committed are assured of safety; therefore they can provide for the security and safety of others. They find in the community sources of lasting significance; therefore, they can accord significance to others, however different from themselves, and can enter into trustful, collaborative relationships wherein the public good and private needs can both contribute to the ultimate decisions. They secure from the community the succorance and support or, to use Hollister's (1967) term, "strens" that must be available if individuals are to cope with inevitable life hazards; therefore they are open to the needs of others and are not walled in by the blinders of local bias or inability to understand the dynamics of community interaction in which they are caught up.

For such people, the community becomes a source of strength. They are aware of and responsive to its dynamics. They move in it with the facility that only self-insight coupled with understanding of the larger dynamics of social organization can engender. They are the cosmopolitans who have not forgotten how to be locals; and they are the locals who know also how to be cosmopolitans. I think the mental health field can help produce such people and the communities that nurture them. It is important to try.

References

Aberle, D., "Introducing Preventive Psychiatry into a Community," *Human Organ.*, **9**, 1950, 5–9.

Aberle, D., and K. Naegele, "Middle-Class Fathers' Occupational Role and Attitudes Toward Children," *Amer. J. Orthopsychiat.*, **22**, 1952, 366–378.

Alinsky, S., *Reveille for Radicals.* Chicago: University of Chicago Press, 1946.

Alinsky, S., "The War on Poverty—Political Pornography," *J. soc. Issues*, **21**, 1965, 41–47.

Altrocchi, J., C. Spielberger, and C. Eisdorfer, "Mental Health Consultation with Groups," *Community ment. Health J.*, **1**, 1965, 127–134.

Bahn, Anita, "An Outline for Community Mental Health Research," *Community ment. Health J.*, **1**, 1965, 23–28.

Baler, L., "Training for Research in Community Mental Health," *Community ment. Health J.*, **3**, 1967, 250–253.

Barker, R., "Explorations in Ecological Psychology," *Amer. Psychologist*, **20**, 1965, 1–14.

Barker, R., and H. Wright, *Midwest and Its Children.* Illinois: Row, Peterson, 1954.

Beiser, M., "Poverty, Social Disintegration, and Personality," *J. soc. Issues*, **21**, 1965, 56–78.

Bellamy, A., "Training for Community Action in an Urban Setting," *Adult Leadership*, **11**, 1962.

Benne, K., "Criteria of a Mature Community, Training Reports and Items No. 120," Boston University Human Relations Center, undated.

Bennett, C. et al., *Community Psychology: a Report of the Boston Conference on the Education of Psychologists for Community Mental Health.* Boston: Boston University and South Shore Mental Health Center, 1966.

Bennis, W., "Leadership and Administrative Behavior: The Problem of Authority," *Admin. Science quart.*, **4**, 1959, 259–301.

Bennis, W., K. Benne, and R. Chin, *The Planning of Change.* New York: Holt, Rinehart, and Winston, 1961.

Biddle, W. and L. Biddle, *The Community Development Process: The Rediscovery of Local Initiative.* New York: Holt, Rinehart, and Winston, 1965.

Bindman, A., "Problems Associated with Community Mental Health Programs," *Community ment. Health J.* **2**, 1966, 333–338.

Blane, H., J. Muller, and M. Chafetz, "Acute Psychiatric Services in the General Hospital: II. Current Status of Emergency Psychiatric Services," *Amer. J. Psychiat.*, **124**, 1967 Suppl., 37–45.

Blum, R. and J. Downing, "Staff Response to Innovation in a Mental Health Service," *Amer. J. Publ. Health*, **54**, 1964, 1230–1240.

Bradford, L., J. Gibb, and K. Benne, *T-Group Theory and Laboratory Method: Innovation in Re-Education*. New York: Wiley, 1964.

Bragg, R., D. Klein, and Elizabeth Lindemann, *Tenth Anniversary Report of the Wellesley Human Relations Service, Inc.* Wellesley: Wellesley Human Relations Service, Inc., 1958.

Brickman, H., "Community Mental Health—the Metropolitan View," *Amer. J. Publ. Health*, **57**, 1967, 641–650.

Brown, B., in C. Dorset (Ed.), *Planning, Programming and Design for the Community Mental Health Center*. New York City: Mental Health Materials Center, 1967

Brownell, B., *The Human Community*. New York: Harper and Bros., 1950.

Bruyn, S., *Human Perspective in Sociology: The Methodology of Participant Observation*. Englewood Cliffs, N.J.: Prentice-Hall, 1966.

Buell, B. et al., *Community Planning for Human Services*. New York: Columbia University Press, 1952.

Burnes, A. and S. Roen, "Social Roles and Adaptation to the Community," *Community ment. Health J.*, **3**, 1967, 153–158.

Calhoun, J., "Population Density and Social Pathology," *Sci. Amer.*, **206**, 1962, 139–146.

Caplan, G., *Concepts of Mental Health and Consultation*. Washington: U. S. Dept. of Health, Education and Welfare, Social Security Administration, Children's Bureau, USGPO, Publication No. 373, 1959.

Caplan, G., *Principles of Preventive Psychiatry*. New York: Basic Books, 1964.

Caplan, G., E. Mason, and D. Kaplan, "Four Studies of Crisis in Parents of Prematures," *Community ment. Health J.*, **1**, 1965, 149–161.

Chapple, E., "Contributions of Anthropology to Institutional Psychiatry," *Human Organ.* **13**, 1955, 11–16.

Chase, S., *Roads to Agreement*. New York: Harper and Bros., 1951.

Clark K., *Social Power and Social Change in Contemporary America*. Washington, D. C.: Equal Employment Opportunity Program, Dept. of State, 1966.

Clausen, J., "Sociology of Mental Disease," in H. Freeman, S. Levine, and L. Reeder, (Eds.), *Handbook of Medical Sociology*, Englewood Cliffs, N.J.: Prentice-Hall, 1963.

Coleman, J. *Community Conflict*. Glencoe, Illinois: The Free Press, 1959.

Coser, L. *The Functions of Social Conflict*. Glencoe, Illinois: The Free Press, 1956.

Counts, G. S., "The Impact of Technological Change," in W. Bennis, K. Benne, and R. Chin (Eds.), *The Planning of Change*, New York: Holt, Rinehart, and Winston, 1961.

Cumming, E. and J. Cumming, *Closed Ranks*. Cambridge: Harvard University Press, 1957.

Daniels, D. and J. Koldau, "Marginal Man, the Tether of Tradition, and Intentional Social System Therapy," *Community ment. Health J.*, **3**, 1967, 13–20.

Dean, J., "Participant Observation and Interviewing," in J. Doby, (Ed.) *An Introduction to Social Research*, Pennsylvania: Stackpole, 1954.

Demone, H., "The Limits of Rationality in Planning," *Community ment. Health J.*, **1**, 1965, 375–382.

Devitt, M. et al., "Survey of Mental Health Problems Encountered in Wellesley by the Various Professions and Agencies in the Month of March," *Human Relations Service*, 1953.

Duhl, L., *The Urban Condition: People and Policy in the Metropolis*. New York: Basic Books, 1963.

Dumont, M., "Tavern Culture: the Sustenance of Homeless Men," *Amer. J. Orthopsy-chiat.*, **37**, 1967, 938–945.

Dunham, H. and S. Weinberg, *The Culture of the State Mental Hospital.* Detroit: Wayne State Univ. Press, 1960.

Fairweather, G., *Methods for Experimental Social Innovation.* New York: Wiley, 1967.

Faris, E. and H. Dunham, *Mental Disorders in Urban Areas.* Chicago: University of Chicago Press, 1939.

Fexil R., "The National Mental Health Program," *Amer. J. Publ. Health,* **54**, 1964, 1804–1809.

Felix, R., "Suicide: a Neglected Problem," *Amer. J. Publ. Health,* **55**, 1965, 16–20.

Franklin, R. (Ed.), *Patterns of Community Development.* Washington: Public Affairs Press, 1966.

Franklin, R., and Paula Franklin, *Urban Decision Making—the Findings from a Conference, Applications of Human Relations Laboratory Training, No. 1,* Washington, D. C.: National Training Laboratories, 1967.

Freeman, L. et al., *Local Community Leadership.* Syracuse, N.Y.: University College of Syracuse, 1960.

Freeman, L. et al., *Metropolitan Decisionmaking: Further Analyses from the Syracuse Study of Local Community Leadership.* Syracuse, N. Y.: University College of Syracuse, 1962.

Fried, M., "Grieving for a Lost Home," in L. Duhl (Ed.), *The Urban Condition,* New York: Basic Books, 1963.

Gans, H., *The Urban Villagers.* Glencoe, Illinois: The Free Press, 1962.

Glidewell, J., "Perspectives in Community Health," in C. Bennett et al. (Eds.), *Community Psychology,* Boston: Boston University and South Shore Mental Health Center, 1966.

Glidewell, J. and L. Stringer, "The Educational Institution and the Health Institution," in E. Bower, and W. Hollister (Eds.), *Behavioral Science Frontiers in Education.* New York: Wiley, 1967.

Goffman, E., *Stigma: Notes on the Management of Spoiled Identity.* Englewood Cliffs, N.J.: Prentice-Hall, 1963.

Goldfarb, A., L. Moses, and J. Downing, "Reliability of Psychiatrists' Ratings in Community Case Finding," *Amer. J. Publ. Health,* **57**, 1967a, 94–106.

Goldfarb, A., L. Moses, J. Downing, and D. Leighton, "Reliability of Newly Trained Raters in Community Case Finding," *Amer. J. Publ. Health,* **57**, 1967b, 2149–2157.

Gordon, C., *The Social System of the High School.* Glencoe, Illinois: The Free Press, 1958.

Gordon, E., "A Review of Programs of Compensatory Education," *Amer. J. Orthopsy-chiat.,* **35**, 1965, 640–657.

Gouldner, A., "Locals and Cosmopolitans: Toward an Analysis of Latent Social Roles, I," *Admin. Sci. quart.,* **2**, 1957, 281–306.

Griffiths, W. and A. Knutson, "The Role of Mass Media in Public Health," *Amer. J. Publ. Health,* **50**, 1960, 515–523.

Gross, N., W. Mason, and A. McEachern, *Explorations in Role Analysis.* New York: Wiley, 1958.

Gruber, S., "The Concept of Task-Orientation in the Analysis of Play Behavior of Children Entering Kindergarten," *Amer. J. Orthopsychiat.,* **24**, 1954, 326–355.

Gruenberg, E. (Ed.), *Evaluating the Effectiveness of Mental Health Services.* New York: Milbank Memorial Fund, 1966.

Guthrie, T., *A Life in the Theatre.* New York: McGraw-Hill, 1959.

Hadley, J. and J. True, "The Associate Degree in Mental Health Technology," *Clin. Psychologist*. In Press.

Hagnell, O., *A Prospective Study of the Incidence of Mental Disorder: the Lundby Project*. Stockholm: Svenska Bokforlaget, Bonniers, Norstedts, 1966.

Hall, E., *The Hidden Dimension*. New York: Doubleday, 1966.

Hallenback, W., "Conflict and Co-operation in American Communities," in C. Mial and D. Mial (Eds.), *Our Community*, New York: New York University Press, 1960.

Hargrove, E., "A State's Perspective in Federal Mental Health Programming," *Amer. J. Publ. Health*, **57**, 1967, 1208–1213.

Herzog, E., *Some Guide Lines for Evaluating Research*. Washington, D.C.: Children's Bureau, 1959.

Hill, R., *Families Under Stress*. New York: Harper and Bros., 1949.

Hoaglund, H. and R. Burhoe, Introduction to the Issue on *Evolution and Man's Progress, Daedalus*, Summer, 1961.

Hobbs, N., "Mental Health's Third Revolution," *Amer. J. Orthopsychiat.*, **34**, 1964, 822–833.

Hollingshead, A. and F. Redlich, *Social Class and Mental Illness*. New York: Wiley, 1958.

Hollister, W., "Some Problems of Strategy in Providing School Mental Health Services," *Amer. J. Publ. Health*, **53**, 1963, 1447–1451.

Hollister, W., "The Concept of 'Strens' in Education: A Challenge to Curriculum Development," in E. Bower, and W. Hollister, *Behavioral Science Frontiers in Education*, New York: Wiley, 1967.

Hughes, C., M. Tremblay, R. Rapaport, and A. Leighton, *People of Cove and Woodlot: Communities from the Viewpoint of Social Psychiatry, Vol. II*. The Stirling County Study of Psychiatric Disorder and Socio-Cultural Environment, New York: Basic Books, 1960.

Hunter, F., *Community Power Structure: A Study of Decision Makers*. Chapel Hill: University of North Carolina Press, 1953.

Jahoda, M. et al., *Research Methods in Social Relations, with Special Reference to Prejudice*. New York: Dryden, 1951.

Jahoda, M., *Current Concepts of Positive Mental Health*. New York: Basic Books, 1958.

James, G. and P. Mico, "Community Study and Leadership: Keys to Effective Health Action," *Amer. J. Publ. Health*, **54**, 1964, 1957–1963.

James, R., "Measures of Effective Community Development: an Appraisal of Community Action as a Social Movement," *Inter. Rev. Community Developm.*, No. 8, 1961, 5–10.

Jenkins, D.H., "Social Engineering in Educational Change: An Outline of Method," *Progressive Educ.* **26**, 1949, 193–197.

Jonassen, C., *Interrelationships Among Dimensions of Community Systems: A Factorial Analysis of Eighty-Two Variables*. Columbus: Ohio State University Press, 1959.

Jones, M., *The Therapeutic Community*. New York: Basic Books, 1953.

Kahn, A., "From Delinquency Treatment to Community Development," in P. Lazarsfeld, W. Sewell, and H. Wilensky, *The Uses of Sociology*, New York: Basic Books, 1967.

Kantor, M., I. Glidewell, I. Mensh, and M. Gildea, "Socio-Economic Level and Maternal Attitude toward Parent-Child Relationship," *Human Organ.*, **16**, 1958, 44–48.

Kaplan, B., R. Reed, and W. Richardson, Jr., "A Comparison of the Incidence of Hospitalized and Non-Hospitalized Cases of Psychosis in Two Communities," *Amer. sociol. Rev.*, **21**, 1956, 472–479.

Kelly, G., *The Psychology of Personal Constructs*. New York: W.W. Norton, 1955.

Kelly, J., "Naturalistic Observations and Theory Confirmation: an Example," *Human Development,* 10, 1967, 212–222.

Kerr, C., "Industrial Conflict and Its Mediation," *Amer. J. Soc.,* 60, 1954, 230–245.

Kevin, D., "Use of the Group Method in Consultation," in Lydia Rapoport (Ed.), *Consultation in Social Work Practice,* New York: National Association of Social Workers, 1963, 69–84.

Klein, D. and Elizabeth Lindemann, "Approaches to Pre-School Screening," *J. School Health,* 34, 1964.

Klein, D. and A. Ross, "Kindergarten Entry: A Study of Role Transition," in M. Krugman (Ed.), *Orthopsychiatry and the School.* New York: Amer. Orthopsychiat. Assoc., 1958, 60–69.

Knight, J., T. Friedman, and J. Sulianti, "Epidemic Hysteria: a Field Study," *Amer. J. Publ. Health,* 55, 1965, 858–865.

Kramer, B., "Tenant Participation in Public Housing," *Community Ment. Health J.,* 3, 1967, 211–215.

Lapouse, R., "Problems in Studying the Prevalence of Psychiatric Disorder," *Amer. J. Publ. Health,* 57, 1967, 947–954.

Leighton, A., *My Name Is Legion. Vol. I,* The Stirling County Study of Psychiatric Disorder and Sociocultural Environment, New York: Basic Books, 1959.

Leighton, A., "Poverty and Social Change," *Sci. Amer.* May 1965.

Leighton, D., "The Distribution of Psychiatric Symptoms in a Small Town," *Amer. J. Psychol.,* 112, 1956, 716–723.

Leighton, D., J. Harding, D. Macklin, A. Macmillan, and A. Leighton, *The Character of Danger: Vol. III,* The Stirling County Study of Psychiatric Disorder and Sociocultural Environment, New York: Basic Books, 1963.

Lemkau, P., C. Tietze, and M. Cooper, "Mental Hygiene Problems in an Urban District, I." *Ment. Hyg.* 25, 1941, 626–646; II, *Ment. Hyg.* 26, 1942; III, *Ment. Hyg.,* 26, 1942; IV, *Ment. Hyg.,* 27, 1943.

Levin, G., "Plan for the Consultation and Education Service of the Sound View Throgs Neck Community Mental Health Center," mimeographed, 1967.

Lewin, K., "Group Decision and Social Change," in T. Newcomb, and E. Hartley (Eds.), *Readings in Social Psychology,* New York: Holt, Rinehart, and Winston, 1947.

Lewin, K., *Resolving Social Conflict.* New York: Harper and Bros., 1958.

Lewis, G., *A Technique in Social Geography for the Delimitation of Residential Sub-Regions.* Unpublished doctoral dissertation, Harvard University, Dept. of Geology, 1956.

Leys, W., *Ethics For Policy Decision.* Englewood Cliffs, N.J.: Prentice-Hall, 1952.

Libo, L. and C. Griffith, "Developing Mental Health Programs in Areas Lacking Professional Facilities: the Community Consultant Approach in New Mexico, *Community ment. Health J.,* 2, 1966, 163–169.

Liebow, E., *Tally's Corner: a Study of Negro Streetcorner Men.* Boston: Little, Brown, 1966.

Lindemann, E. C., *The Community—An Introduction to the Study of Community Leadership and Organization.* New York: Association Press, 1921.

Lindemann, Elizabeth, J. Rosenblith, W. Allinsmith, L. Budd, and S. Shapiro, "Predicting School Adjustment before Entry," *J. sch. Psychol.,* 6, 1967, 24–42.

Lindemann, Erich, "Symptomatology and Management of Acute Grief," *Amer. J. Psych.,* 101, 1944, 141–148.

Lindemann, Erich, "Modifications in the Course of Ulcerative Colitis in Relationship to Changes in Life Situations and Reaction Patterns," in *Life Stress and Bodily*

Diseases, **29,** 1950, 706–723, Association for Research in Nervous and Mental Diseases.

Lindemann, Erich, "The Wellesley Project for the Study of Certain Problems in Community Mental Health," in *Interrelations between the Social Environment and Psychiatric Disorders,* New York: Milbank Memorial Fund, 1953, 165–185.

Lindemann, Erich, "Mental Health—Fundamental to a Dynamic Epidemiology of Health," in I. Galdston (Ed.), *The Epidemiology of Health,* New York: Health Education Council, 1953, 109–123.

Lindemann, Erich, "The Meaning of Crisis in Individual and Family Living," *Teachers Coll. Rec.,* **57,** No. 4, 1956.

Lindemann, Erich, and A. Ross, "A Follow-up Study of a Predictive Test of Social Adaptation in Pre-School Children," in G. Caplan (Ed.), *Emotional Problems of Early Childhood,* New York: Basic Books, 1955.

Lindemann, Erich, W. Vaughan, and M. McGinnis, "Preventive Intervention in a Four-Year-Old Child Whose Father Committed Suicide," in G. Caplan (Ed.), *Emotional Problems of Early Childhood,* New York: Basic Books, 1955.

Lippitt, R., "The Effects of Authoritarian and External Controls on the Development of Mental Health," in R. Ojemann (Ed.), *Recent Research on Creative Approaches to Environmental Stress,* Ames, Iowa: State University of Iowa, 1965.

Lippitt, R., "The Use of Social Research to Improve Social Practice," *Amer. J. Orthopsychiat.,* **35,** 1965, 663–669.

Lippitt, R., J. Watson, and B. Westley, *The Dynamics of Planned Change.* New York: Harcourt Brace, 1958.

Loomis, C., *Social Systems.* New York: Van Nostrand, 1960.

Lowry, R., *Who's Running This Town.* New York: Harper and Row, 1965.

McGinnis, M., "The Wellesley Project Program of Pre-School Emotional Assessment," *J. psychiat. soc. Work,* **23,** 1954, 135–141.

McMahon, B. et al., *Epidemiologic Methods.* Boston: Little, Brown, 1960.

McNeil, E., "Analysis of an Ailing Monster: School Organization," in E. Bower, and W. Hollister, *Behavioral Science Frontiers of Education.* New York: Wiley, 1967.

Mead, G., *Mind, Self, and Society.* Chicago: University of Chicago Press, 1934.

Menninger, K., M. Mayman, and P. Preger, "The Urge to Classify," in R. Dentler, *Major American Social Problems,* Chicago: Rand McNally, 1967.

Mial, D. and H. C. Mial, "Leadership Training," *Nat. civic Rev.* May 1962, 257–262.

Mial, D. and H. C. Mial, *Our Community.* New York: New York University Press, 1960.

Mial, H. C., "Community Development—a Democratic Social Process," *Adult Leadership,* April 1958, 277–282.

Mial, H. C., "Models of Community Action," in H. C. Mial, and D. Mial (Eds.), *Forces in Community Development, Selected Reading Series No. 4,* Washington: National Training Laboratories, National Education Association, 1961.

Milbank Memorial Fund. *Interrelation between the Social Environment and Psychiatric Disorders.* New York: Milbank Memorial Fund, 1953.

Miller, D., *Worlds that Fail. Part I: a Retrospective Analysis of Mental Patients' Careers.* Sacramento: California Dept. of Mental Hygiene, Bureau of Research, 1965.

Moe, E., "Consulting with a Community System: a Case Study," *J. Soc. Issues,* **15,** 1959, 28–35.

Moore, B. Jr., "Sociological Theory and Contemporary Politics," *Amer. J. Soc.,* **61,** 1955, 107–115.

Muller, J., M. Chafetz, and H. Blane, "Acute Psychiatric Services in the General Hospital: III Statistical Survey," *Amer. J. Psychiat.,* **124,** Oct. 1967 Suppl., 46–57.

Mumford, L., *The Culture of Cities.* New York: Harcourt Brace, 1938.

Naegele, K., "A Mental Health Project in a Boston Suburb," in B. Paul (Ed.), *Health, Culture, and Community: Case Studies of Public Reactions to Health Programs,* New York: Russell Sage, 1955.

Nehru, J., *The Discovery of India.* New York: John Day, 1946.

Nelson, B., "Community—Dreams and Realities," in C. Friedrich (Ed.), *Community,* New York: Liberal Arts, 1959.

Nelson, L. et al., *Community Structure and Change.* New York: Macmillan, 1960.

Newton, R. and R. Brown, "A Preventive Approach to Developmental Problems in School Children," in E. Bower, and W. Hollister (Eds.), *Behavioral Science Frontiers in Education,* New York: Wiley, 1967.

Osterweil, J., "School Psychology and Comprehensive Community Mental Health Planning," *Community ment. Health J.,* **2,** 1966, 129–133.

Ozarin, L., The Community Mental Health Center—a Public Health Facility, *Amer. J. Publ. Health,* **56,** 1966, 26–31.

Parad, H. (Ed.), *Crisis Intervention: Selected Readings.* New York: Family Service Association of America, 1965.

Peck, H., S. Kaplan, and M. Roman, "Prevention, Treatment, and Social Action: a Strategy of Intervention in a Disadvantaged Urban Area," *Amer. J. Orthopsychiat.,* **36,** 1966, 57–69.

Phillips, B., *Social Research Strategy and Tactics.* New York: Macmillan, 1966.

Phillips, D., "The 'True Prevalence' of Mental Illness in a New England State," *Community ment. Health J.,* **2,** 1966, 35–40.

Phillips, L., "The Competence Criterion for Mental Health Programs," *Community ment. Health J.,* **3,** 1967, 73–76.

Plunkett, R. and J. Gordon, *Epidemiology and Mental Illness.* New York: Basic Books. 1960.

Poston, R., *Democracy Is You.* New York: Harper, 1953.

Pratt, S. and J. Tooley, "Human Actualization Teams: the Perspective of Contract Psychology," *Amer. J. Orthopsychiat.,* **36,** 1966, 881–895.

Reiff, R. and F. Riessman, "The Indigenous Non-Professional: a Strategy of Change in Community Action and Community Mental Health Programs," *Community ment. Health J., Monograph No.* 1, 1965.

Rhodes, W., "Psychosocial Learning," in E. Bower, and W. Hollister (Eds.), *Behavioral Science Frontiers in Education,* New York: Wiley, 1967.

Rice, E. and S. Krakow, "Hospitalization of a Parent for Mental Illness: a Crisis for Children," *Amer. J. Orthopsychiat.,* **36,** 1966, 868–872.

Rieman, D., "Group Mental Health Consultation with Public Health Nurses," in Lydia Rapoport (Ed.), *Consultation in Social Work Practice,* New York: National Association of Social Workers, 1963, 85–98.

Riessman, F., J. Cohen, and A. Pearl (Eds.), *Mental Health of the Poor.* Illinois: The Free Press, 1964.

Riessman, F., and S. Scribner, "The Under-utilization of Mental Health Services by Workers and Low-Income Groups: Causes and Cures," *Amer. J. Psychiat.,* **121,** 1965, 798–801.

Robinson, R., "A Report on the Project on Community Resources in Mental Health," *Amer. J. Publ. Health,* **53,** 1963, 609–614.

Rosenberg, P. and M. Fuller, "Human Relations Seminar: a Group Work Experiment in Nursing Education," *Ment. Hyg.*, **39**, 1955, 406–432.

Rosenblum, G. and L. Hassol, "Training for New Mental Health Roles," *Ment. Hyg.*, **52**, 1968, 45–56.

Rosenblum, G. and D. Ottenstein, "From Child Guidance to Community Mental Health: Problems in Transition," *Community ment. Health J.*, **1**, 1965, 276–283.

Ross, M., *Community Organization*. New York: Harper and Bros., 1955.

Ross, M., *Case Histories in Community Organization*. New York: Harper and Bros., 1958.

Ruesch, J. and G. Bateson, *Communication, the Social Matrix of Psychiatry*. New York: Norton, 1951.

Sanders, I., *The Community: An Introduction to a Social System*. New York: Ronald, 1958.

Schein, E. and W. Bennis, *Personal and Organizational Change through Group Methods*. New York: Wiley, 1965.

Schwartz, D., "Integration of Hospital and Community Mental Health Services on a County and Regional Basis," *Amer. J. Publ. Health*, **55**, 1965, 873–878.

Seeley, J., R. Sim, and E. Loosley, *Crestwood Heights*. New York: Basic Books, 1956.

Selltiz, C. et al., *Research Methods in Social Relations*, Rev. Ed. New York: Holt, Rinehart, and Winston, 1959.

Shneidman, E. and N. Farberow, "The Los Angeles Suicide Prevention Center: a Demonstration of Public Health Feasibilities," *Amer. J. Publ. Health*, **55**, 1965, 21–26.

Solnit, A., The Psychiatric Council: Applied Psychiatry in an Anti-Poverty Program, *Amer. J. Orthopsychiat.*, **37**, 1967, 495–506.

Sower, C. et al., *Community Involvement*. Glencoe, Illinois: The Free Press, 1957.

Spengler, J. and D. Duncan (Eds.), *Demographic Analysis: Selected Readings*. Glencoe, Illinois: The Free Press, 1956.

Srole, L. et al., *Mental Health in the Metropolis*. New York City: McGraw-Hill Book Co., 1962.

Straus, R. and J. Clausen, "Health, Society, and Social Science," *Ann. Amer. Acad. polit. and soc. Sci.*, **346**, 1963, 1–8.

Thelen, H., *The Dynamics of Groups at Work*. Chicago: University of Chicago Press, 1954.

Thoma, L. and E. Lindemann, "Newcomers' Problems in a Suburban Community," *J. Amer. Inst. Planners*, **27**, 1961, 185–193.

Van Amerongen, T. Suzanne, "Initial Psychiatric Family Studies," *Amer. J. Orthopsychiat.*, **24**, 1954, 73–84.

Vaughan, W. and Emillie Faber, "Field Methods and Techniques—The Systematic Observation of Kindergarten Children," *Human Organ.*, **11**, 1952, 33–36.

Viguers, R., "Who's On Top? Who Knows?" *Mod. Hosp.*, June 1956.

Warren, R., *The Community in America*. Chicago: Rand McNally, 1963.

Warren R., "The Interaction of Community Decision Organizations: Some Basic Concepts and Needed Research," *Soc. Serv. Rev.*, **41**, 1967, 261–270.

Warren, R., "Toward a Reformulation of Community Theory," *Human Organ.*, **15**, 1956.

Warren, R., "Types of Purposive Social Change at the Community Level," Brandeis University Publications in Social Welfare, no. 11, 1965.

Weber, M. *Essays In Sociology*. New York: Oxford University Press, 1946.

Whyte, W., *Organization Man*. New York: Simon and Schuster, 1956.

Wirth, L., *Community Life and Social Policy.* Chicago: University of Chicago Press, 1956.

Yablonski, L., *The Tunnel Back: Synanon.* New York: Macmillan, 1965.

Yolles, S., "Community Appraisal of Mental Health Practices," *Amer. J. Publ. Health,* **54,** 1967, 1970–1976.

Index